Degenerative Spinal Deformity: Creating Lordosis in the Lumbar Spine

Editors

SIGURD BERVEN
PRAVEEN V. MUMMANENI

NEUROSURGERY CLINICS OF NORTH AMERICA

www.neurosurgery.theclinics.com

Consulting Editors
RUSSELL R. LONSER
DANIEL K. RESNICK

July 2018 • Volume 29 • Number 3

ELSEVIER

1600 John F. Kennedy Boulevard • Suite 1800 • Philadelphia, Pennsylvania, 19103-2899

http://www.theclinics.com

NEUROSURGERY CLINICS OF NORTH AMERICA Volume 29, Number 3
July 2018 ISSN 1042-3680, ISBN-13: 978-0-323-64107-4

Editor: Stacy Eastman
Developmental Editor: Laura Fisher

Neurosurgery Clinics of North America (ISSN 1042-3680) is published quarterly by Elsevier Inc., 360 Park Avenue South, New York, NY 10010-1710. Months of issue are January, April, July, and October. Business and Editorial Offices: 1600 John F. Kennedy Blvd., Suite 1800, Philadelphia, PA 19103-2899. Customer Service Office: 11830 Westline Industrial Drive, St. Louis, MO 63146. Periodicals postage paid at New York, NY, and additional mailing offices. Subscription prices are $417.00 per year (US individuals), $711.00 per year (US institutions), $449.00 per year (Canadian individuals), $884.00 per year (Canadian institutions), $505.00 per year (international individuals), $884.00 per year (international institutions), $100.00 per year (US students), and $255.00 per year (international and Canadian students). International air speed delivery is included in all *Clinics* subscription prices. All prices are subject to change without notice. **POSTMASTER:** Send address changes to *Neurosurgery Clinics of North America*, Elsevier Periodicals Customer Service, 11830 Westline Industrial Drive, St. Louis, MO 63146. **Customer Service: 1-800-654-2452 (US and Canada). From outside the US and Canada, call: 1-314-453-7041. Fax: 1-314-453-5170. E-mail: JournalsCustomerService-usa@elsevier.com (for print support) and journalsonlinesupport-usa@elsevier.com (for online support).**

Reprints. For copies of 100 or more, of articles in this publication, please contact the Commercial Reprints Department, Elsevier Inc., 360 Park Avenue South, New York, NY 10010-1710. Tel. 212-633-3874; Fax: 212-633-3820; E-mail: reprints@elsevier.com.

Neurosurgery Clinics of North America is covered in *MEDLINE/PubMed (Index Medicus), EMBASE/Excerpta Medica, and Current Contents/Clinical Medicine (CC/CM).*

Contributors

CONSULTING EDITORS

RUSSELL R. LONSER, MD
Professor and Chair, Department of
Neurological Surgery, The Ohio State
University Wexner Medical Center, Columbus,
Ohio

DANIEL K. RESNICK, MD, MS
Professor and Vice Chairman, Program
Director, Department of Neurosurgery,
University of Wisconsin-Madison School of
Medicine and Public Health, Madison,
Wisconsin

EDITORS

SIGURD BERVEN, MD
Professor in Residence, Chief of
Orthopaedic Spine Service, Department of
Orthopaedic Surgery, University of California,
San Francisco Spine Center, San Francisco,
California

PRAVEEN V. MUMMANENI, MD
Joan O'Reilly Endowed Professor, Vice Chair,
UCSF Neurosurgery, Co-director, University of
California, San Francisco Spine Center,
San Francisco, California

AUTHORS

NEEL ANAND, MD
Professor of Orthopaedics, Department of
Orthopaedic Surgery, Director of Spine
Trauma, Spine Center, Cedars-Sinai Medical
Center, Los Angeles, California

SIGURD BERVEN, MD
Professor in Residence, Chief of
Orthopaedic Spine Service, Department of
Orthopaedic Surgery, University of California,
San Francisco Spine Center, San Francisco,
California

ROBERT M. BRENNER, MS, MD
Department of Orthopaedic Surgery, University
of Minnesota, Minneapolis, Minnesota

PETER G. CAMPBELL, MD
Spine Institute of Louisiana, Shreveport,
Louisiana

PAUL C. CELESTRE, MD
Assistant Professor, The University of
Queensland Medical School, Ochsner Clinic,
New Orleans, Louisiana

ANDREW K. CHAN, MD
Department of Neurosurgery, University of
California, San Francisco, San Francisco,
California

DEAN CHOU, MD
Professor, Department of Neurosurgery,
University of California, San Francisco,
San Francisco, California

WINWARD CHOY, MD
Department of Neurosurgery, University of
California, San Francisco, San Francisco,
California

ANTHONY M. DiGIORGIO, DO, MHA
Resident, Department of Neurosurgery,
Louisiana State University Health Sciences
Center, New Orleans, Louisiana

JOHN R. DIMAR II, MD
Clinical Professor, Department of Orthopaedic
Surgery, University of Louisville School of
Medicine, Norton Leatherman Spine Center,
Louisville, Kentucky

ROBERT K. EASTLACK, MD
Scripps Clinic, San Diego Center for Spinal Disorders, La Jolla, California

CALEB S. EDWARDS, BA
Medical Student, School of Medicine, University of California, San Francisco, San Francisco, California

ANDREW A. FANOUS, MD
Spine Fellow, Department of Neurological Surgery, University of Miami, Miami, Florida

KAI-MING FU, MD
Assistant Professor, Department of Neurosurgery, Weill Cornell Medical College, New York, New York

STEVEN D. GLASSMAN, MD
Professor, Department of Orthopaedic Surgery, University of Louisville School of Medicine, Norton Leatherman Spine Center, Louisville, Kentucky

MUNISH C. GUPTA, MD
Mildred B. Simon Distinguished Professor of Orthopaedic Surgery, Professor of Neurological Surgery, Chief of Pediatric and Adult Spinal Surgery, Co-director of Pediatric and Adult Spinal Deformity Service, Washington University School of Medicine in St. Louis, St Louis, Missouri

SACHIN GUPTA, BS
Department of Orthopaedic Surgery, The George Washington University, Washington, DC

RANDALL J. HLUBEK, MD
Scripps Clinic, San Diego Center for Spinal Disorders, La Jolla, California; Division of Neurosurgery, Barrow Neurological Institute, Phoenix, Arizona

RYAN J. HOEL, MD
Department of Orthopaedic Surgery, University of Minnesota, Minneapolis, Minnesota

ADAM S. KANTER, MD
Department of Neurological Surgery, University of Pittsburgh Medical Center, Pittsburgh, Pennsylvania

ISAAC O. KARIKARI, MD
Assistant Professor of Neurosurgery and Orthopedic Surgery, Department of Neurosurgery, Duke University Medical Center, Durham, North Carolina

CHRISTOPHER KONG, MD
Spine Surgeon, Department of Orthopaedic Surgery, Cedars-Sinai Medical Center, Los Angeles, California

RONALD A. LEHMAN, MD
Department of Orthopaedic Surgery, Columbia University Medical Center, The Spine Hospital at NewYork-Presbyterian, New York, New York

LAWRENCE G. LENKE, MD
Department of Orthopaedic Surgery, Columbia University Medical Center, The Spine Hospital at NewYork-Presbyterian, New York, New York

JASON I. LIOUNAKOS, MD
Resident, Department of Neurological Surgery, University of Miami, Miami, Florida

JOSEPH M. LOMBARDI, MD
Department of Orthopaedic Surgery, Columbia University Medical Center, The Spine Hospital at NewYork-Presbyterian, New York, New York

LIONEL N. METZ, MD
Assistant Professor, Department of Orthopedic Surgery, University of California, San Francisco, San Francisco, California

CATHERINE A. MILLER, MD
Fellow, Department of Neurosurgery, University of California, San Francisco, San Francisco, California

PRAVEEN V. MUMMANENI, MD
Joan O'Reilly Endowed Professor, Vice Chair, UCSF Neurosurgery, Co-director, University of California, San Francisco Spine Center, San Francisco, California

GREGORY M. MUNDIS Jr, MD
Scripps Clinic, San Diego Center for Spinal Disorders, La Jolla, California

PIERCE D. NUNLEY, MD
Spine Institute of Louisiana, Shreveport, Louisiana

TAEMIN OH, MD
Department of Neurosurgery, University of California, San Francisco, San Francisco, California

JASON PALUZZI, MD
Department of Neurosurgery and Brain Repair, University of South Florida, Tampa, Florida

PAUL PARK, MD
Professor, Department of Neurosurgery, University of Michigan, Ann Arbor, Michigan

DAVID W. POLLY Jr, MD
Professor and Chief of Spine Surgery, Department of Orthopaedic Surgery, University of Minnesota, Minneapolis, Minnesota

CHRISTOPHER I. SHAFFREY, MD, FACS
Department of Neurological Surgery, University of Virginia, Charlottesville, Virginia

JAMAL N. SHILLINGFORD, MD
Department of Orthopaedic Surgery, Columbia University Medical Center, The Spine Hospital at NewYork-Presbyterian, New York, New York

JUAN S. URIBE, MD
Department of Neurological Surgery, Barrow Neurological Institute, St. Joseph's Hospital and Medical Center, Chief, Division of Spinal Disorders, Volker K.H. Sonntag Chair of Spine Research, St. Joseph's Hospital and Medical Center, Phoenix, Arizona

MICHAEL S. VIRK, MD, PhD
Assistant Professor, Department of Neurosurgery, Weill Cornell Medical College, NewYork-Presbyterian, New York, New York

RISHI WADHWA, MD
Assistant Professor, Neurosurgery, University of California, San Francisco Spine Center, San Francisco, California

MICHAEL Y. WANG, MD
Professor, Department of Neurological Surgery, University of Miami, Miami, Florida

DAVID S. XU, MD
Department of Neurological Surgery, Barrow Neurological Institute, St. Joseph's Hospital and Medical Center, Phoenix, Arizona

Contents

Preop Planning and Goals of Surgery

Pelvic incidence defines the amount of lordosis required in the lumbar spine, and a lumbar lordosis within 11° of the pelvic incidence defines alignment of the lumbo-pelvic region. Pelvic tilt is a compensatory mechanism that allows patients to achieve sagittal balance in the setting of decreased lumbar lordosis with the primary compensatory mechanisms being hip extension and knee flexion. Planning an adult lumbar deformity operation requires a comprehensive history and physical examination and thorough radiographic evaluation with the goal of restoring alignment between the pelvic incidence and lumbar lordosis and restoring a normal pelvic tilt.

Alignment of the lumbar spine has an important impact on the segmental motion, degenerative pathology, and health-related quality of life. The relationship between lumbar lordosis and pelvic incidence is predictive in the pathogenesis of spinal disorders, including disk degeneration, spondylolisthesis, and adjacent segment degeneration. This article reviews the relationship between lumbar and pelvic alignment with pathology of the lumbar spine, provides goals for appropriate alignment in reconstructive surgery, and discusses strategies for effective realignment of the spine.

Open Surgical Techniques

Restoration of physiologic lumbar lordosis is a fundamental principle of spinal deformity surgery. Techniques using multilevel anterior lumbar interbody fusion or pedicle subtraction osteotomy (PSO) are described. Multilevel anterior lumbar interbody fusion provides a gradual multilevel correction and avoids the morbidity associated with PSO but necessitates familiarity with the anterior approach or an approach surgeon. PSO provides a large angular correction at a single level, requires only one approach, and allows for simultaneous multiplanar correction and open posterior decompression. This article provides guidance on the appropriate use of each technique for restoration of lumbar lordosis in patients with degenerative lumbar deformity.

In adult spinal deformity, the pedicle subtraction osteotomy is a useful technique to provide correction, especially in rigid, previously fused spines. However, it is not without complications. In an effort to prevent pseudoarthrosis, a new technique using 4 rods has been pioneered to decrease stress on the 2 long rods while allowing for maintenance of correction with 2 smaller rods. One should also use careful neuromonitoring, especially during closure, to be able to make adjustments in time to prevent the development of neurologic deficits. Nevertheless, significant correction can be achieved and patients' functional outcomes can be greatly improved.

The increase in the aging population has led to an overall increase in the number of elderly patients undergoing spinal fusion surgery. This patient population, however, exhibits significant treatment challenges because of poor bone quality. By virtue of exhibiting decreased pullout strength and insertional torque, osteoporotic patients are at a substantial risk of developing vertebral fractures, instrumentation failure, pseudoarthrosis, and proximal junctional failures. It is, therefore, imperative for the treating surgeon to optimize bone health before recommending a spinal fusion surgery. Several preoperative medical therapies (vitamin D, calcium, bisphosphonates, parathyroid hormone, and so forth) exist to optimize bone health.

High-grade dysplastic spondylolisthesis (HGDS) is a subset of L5-S1 spondylolisthesis that occurs due to dysmorphic anatomy at the lumbosacral junction, often resulting in sagittal imbalance. Enhanced understanding of global sagittal alignment has led many to preferentially treat HGDS with reduction and fusion to restore sagittal balance. This article reviews published surgical techniques for obtaining sagittal correction in HGDS and evaluates the current evidence regarding the associated surgical complications.

The indications for sacropelvic fixation continue to evolve with emerging instrumentation technologies and advancing techniques. Common indications include long construct fusions, high-grade spondylolisthesis, sacral fractures, sacral tumors, and global sagittal and/or coronal imbalance, among others. The authors' preferred technique is through use of a freehand S2-alar-iliac screw placement.

MIS Surgical Techniques

Minimally invasive surgery (MIS) is an alternative to open surgery for adult spinal deformity correction. However, not all patients are ideal candidates for MIS correction. The minimally invasive spinal deformity surgery algorithm is a systematic and reproducible decision-making framework for surgeons to identify patients appropriate for deformity correction by MIS techniques. Key spinopelvic parameters, including sagittal vertical axis, pelvic tilt, pelvic incidence to lumbar lordosis mismatch, and coronal Cobb angle, are used to guide surgeons toward 3 treatment classes ranging from MIS to traditional open approaches. This article updates the minimally invasive spinal deformity surgery algorithm and presents representative cases.

The transpsoas approach is a powerful tool in correcting adult spinal deformity secondary to the degenerative process. It may be used as a stand-alone construct or in combination with other approaches to correct both coronal and sagittal malalignment. Preoperative planning with careful analysis of full-length 36-in radiographs and an MRI of the lumbar spine is essential in determining the safety and feasibility of this approach. Ultimately the goals of deformity correction must be achieved, and lateral lumbar interbody fusion is a valuable tool that can aid in achieving these goals while minimizing perioperative morbidity.

The prepsoas oblique approach to the lumbar spine provides many similar benefits of the transpsoas lateral approach. Because the psoas is not traversed, however, many of the postoperative complications associated with psoas violation are reduced. Working at an oblique angle to the spine can be challenging, and the approach may be unfamiliar for the surgeon. This article provides a technical description and nuances of the approach.

Lateral anterior column release (ACR) is a powerful extension of the minimally invasive lateral lumbar interbody fusion procedure that incorporates division of the anterior longitudinal ligament to allow manipulation of the anterior and middle spinal columns. The resulting surgical control permits restoration of significant segmental lordosis that, when combined with varying posterior column releases, can achieve global sagittal realignment on par with traditional 3-column osteotomies. As a result, ACR is a factor in the growth of minimally invasive strategies for the correction of spinal deformities.

Surgical correction of deformity is a complex endeavor. Although more traditional, open techniques remain important, minimally invasive surgery (MIS) techniques have been increasingly studied as an alternative approach. In particular, the circumferential MIS approach, which may incorporate a lateral/anterior as well as a subsequent posterior approach, has been investigated as a promising algorithm/protocol. Utilization of navigation guidance during MIS deformity correction is an important intraoperative tool for the surgeon.

The transforaminal lumbar interbody fusion (TLIF) is a well-established 3-column fusion technique that can be used to manage lumbar stenosis, instability, and deformity. Having been in use for more than 20 years, it has evolved into many different renditions, including protocols using minimally invasive surgery (MIS) approaches. To avoid the development of flatback syndrome, it is important that a TLIF procedural technique is capable of reproducibly restoring lordosis. This article describes one of many MIS TLIF protocols and presents some of its previously published outcomes.

For patients with significant spinal deformity, the pedicle subtraction osteotomy provides a powerful means for correction, albeit with high morbidity. With the trend toward minimally invasive spine surgery, multiple less invasive techniques have been devised; however, there seems to be an upper limit to the degree of correction possible. The mini–open pedicle subtraction osteotomy addresses these limitations by minimizing the extent of soft tissue destruction needed to perform the osteotomy and by using the rod-cantilever technique to achieve maximum lordosis. Preliminary data are promising, with significant improvements in patient-reported clinical outcome measures as well as coronal and sagittal alignment.

Adult degenerative scoliosis treatment is complicated by its predilection for an elderly patient population that often exhibits multiple unrelated medical comorbidities. As spine surgeons attempt to treat this disease process with less invasive solutions, the fractional curve at L4, L5, and S1 is often overlooked or undertreated secondary to required increased perioperative morbidity associated with its treatment. A treatment strategy to identify, address, and treat the fractional curve with either open or minimally invasive techniques can lead to improved patient outcomes and decreased revision rates in this complicated pathologic process.

NEUROSURGERY CLINICS OF NORTH AMERICA

THE CLINICS ARE AVAILABLE ONLINE!
Access your subscription at:
www.theclinics.com

NEUROSURGERY CLINICS OF NORTH AMERICA

FORTHCOMING ISSUE

October 2018
Coagulation and Hematology in Neurological Surgery
Shahid M. Nimjee and Russell R. Lonser, Editors

January 2019
Low-Grade Glioma
Guy McKhann II and Hugues Duffau, Editor

April 2019
Neuromodulation
Wendell B. Lake, Ashwini D. Sharan, and Chengyuan Wu, Editors

RECENT ISSUES

April 2018
Neurocritical Care
Alejandro A. Rabinstein, Editor

January 2018
Cervical Myelopathy
Michael G. Fehlings, Editor

October 2017
Intraoperative Imaging
Bradley Elder and Ganesh Rao, Editors

RELATED INTEREST

Magnetic Resonance Imaging Clinics August 2016 (Vol. 24, Issue 3)
Update on Spine Imaging
Mario Muto, Editor
Available at: http://www.mri.theclinics.com

Preface

Degenerative Spinal Deformity: Creating Lordosis in the Lumbar Spine

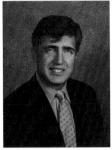
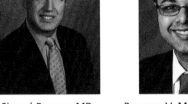

Sigurd Berven, MD   Praveen V. Mummaneni, MD

Editors

Degenerative spinal deformity encompasses a broad range of spectrum of pathologies resulting in the common presentation of malalignment of the spine with clinical presentation of pain, functional limitations, and neural compromise. The operative management of degenerative spinal deformity has the goal of realignment of the spinal column, decompression of the neural elements, and improvement of pain, function, and health-related quality of life. Creating lordosis in the lumbar spine is an important goal of reconstructive surgery in degenerative spinal deformity, and the community of surgeons treating patients recognizes the importance of restoring physiologic lordosis in the lumbar spine in order to avoid adjacent segment pathology and junctional kyphosis and to improve the health status of patients presenting with symptomatic deformity. The techniques of restoring lordosis in reconstructive surgery encompass anterior and posterior approaches to the spine, open surgical approaches and minimally invasive approaches, and techniques and technologies that continue to evolve. There is significant variability in the surgical approaches to degenerative spinal deformity, and the presence of variability is a clear reflection of the absence of a single, evidence-based approach to care. Matching the appropriate surgical approach and technique to the specific indications of a patient is an important goal of optimal care for patients with spinal deformity.

The purpose of this issue is to review the importance of restoration of appropriate alignment of the lumbar spine, and the lumbopelvic junction in reconstructive surgery, and to provide detailed descriptions of surgical techniques, and limitations, for reconstructive surgery by experts from fields of neurosurgery and orthopedic surgery.

The operative management of patients with deformity of the spine is a challenge and is evolving with the development of new techniques and technologies. Approaches to management of patients with spinal deformity are characterized by significant variability between and within subspecialties. The development of an evidence-based approach to the management of spinal deformity requires ongoing critical assessment of clinical outcomes and ongoing collaboration and communication between all physicians who care for patients with disorders of the spine. In this issue, we introduce the importance of lumbopelvic parameters, and the association between lumbopelvic parameters and health status, and why restoration of lumbopelvic parameters is a priority for optimal care of patients with degenerative deformity. The issue is divided into 2 major parts: open surgical approaches to spinal reconstruction and minimally invasive approaches. In the open surgical approaches, techniques, including anterior lumbar interbody fusion, pedicle subtraction osteotomy, reduction of spondylolisthesis, and lumbopelvic fixation, are detailed.

Neurosurg Clin N Am 29 (2018) xiii–xiv
https://doi.org/10.1016/j.nec.2018.04.001
1042-3680/18/© 2018 Published by Elsevier Inc.

Each article emphasizes the advantages and limitations of the open approaches to care, with an emphasis on complication avoidance. The articles on minimally invasive approaches to deformity introduce an algorithm for the management of degenerative deformity in the spine using minimally invasive approaches. The section then details the advantages and limitations of posterior-based interbody, direct lateral and prepsoas approaches to the spine, and new technologies, including image guidance and navigation in reconstructive surgery.

Our goal in this issue is to instruct the reader on the goals of reconstruction in the spine affected by degenerative spinal deformity, with an emphasis on restoring lumbar lordosis and lumbopelvic parameters. The issue includes detailed information on specific techniques, including advantages and limitations of open and minimally invasive approaches. By providing information on contemporary approaches to degenerative spinal deformity, we intend to provide evidence to guide optimal care of patients and to improve the value of surgery for each patient.

Sigurd Berven, MD
Orthopaedic Spine Service
Department of Orthopaedic Surgery
University of California, San Francisco
500 Parnassus Avenue, MU320W
San Francisco, CA 94143-0728, USA

Praveen V. Mummaneni, MD
UCSF Neurosurgery
UCSF Spine Center
505 Parnassus Avenue, M780
San Francisco, CA 94143-0112, USA

E-mail addresses:
Bervens@orthosurg.ucsf.edu (S. Berven)
Praveen.Mummaneni@ucsf.edu
(P.V. Mummaneni)

Spinopelvic Parameters: Lumbar Lordosis, Pelvic Incidence, Pelvic Tilt, and Sacral Slope
What Does a Spine Surgeon Need to Know to Plan a Lumbar Deformity Correction?

Paul C. Celestre, MD[a],*, John R. Dimar II, MD[b], Steven D. Glassman, MD[b]

KEYWORDS

- Lumbar deformity • Lumbar lordosis • Pelvic incidence • Pelvic tilt • Sacral slope
- Pelvic parameters • Sagittal balance

KEY POINTS

- A thorough history and physical examination are essential to successfully treat patients with lumbar spinal deformity.
- In younger patients without spinal deformity, lumbar lordosis (LL) should be within 11° of pelvic incidence (PI).
- A normal pelvic tilt is less than 15°.
- PI-LL mismatch of greater than 11° and a pelvic tilt of greater than 22° is strongly correlated with an Oswestry Disability Index score greater than 40.
- Increasing pelvic tilt is a limited compensatory mechanism to maintain normal sagittal balance in the setting of PI-LL mismatch.

INTRODUCTION AND HISTORICAL CONTEXT

Observations of spinal deformity date to antiquity. Hippocrates described both the normal contours of the spine as well as deformities of the spine and their causes, grouping abnormal spinal alignments under the umbrella term *scoliosis*.[1] Galen of Pergamum defined the terms *kyphosis*, *scoliosis*, and *lordosis*; their use continues as Galen described them to this day.[1] In 1935 Bohler[2] described compensatory mechanisms, including pelvic retroversion, for maintaining an upright posture in patients with posttraumatic kyphosis.[2]

Beginning in the 1970s, the investigations of multiple French surgeons led to a renewed interest in spinal balance.[3,4] Building on this, Jean Dubousset and colleagues[5] introduced the postural cone of economy that highlighted the

Disclosure Statement: Nothing to disclose (P. Celestre). Medronic: consulting, royalties; Norton Hospital: speaking, research funding; DePuy: consulting; Scoliosis Research Society: board member, Education Council Chair; Federation of Spine Associations: board member (J.R. Dimar). Medronic: intellectual property royalties, consulting; Scoliosis Research Society: board member (S.D. Glassman).
[a] Department of Orthopaedic Surgery, University of Queensland Medical School, Ochsner Clinic, 1514 Jefferson Highway, New Orleans, LA 70121, USA; [b] Department of Orthopaedic Surgery, University of Louisville School of Medicine, Norton Leatherman Spine Center, 210 East Gray Street, Suite 900, Louisville, KT 40202, USA
* Corresponding author.
E-mail address: paul.celestre@ochsner.org

neurosurgery.theclinics.com

importance of the maintenance of upright posture with minimal physical effort. Duval-Beaupère,[6] and later Jackson and Hales,[7] quantified sagittal measurements of the pelvis, including pelvic retroversion, LL, and sagittal alignment, establishing the pelvis as central to global sagittal balance and PI the primary determinant of lordosis in a well-aligned lumbo-pelvic region.

In 2005, Glassman and colleagues[8] demonstrated that positive sagittal balance directly correlates with patient-reported self-assessment measures, specifically that increasing positive sagittal imbalance was directly related to worsening symptoms. Lafage and colleagues[9] further refined

this idea, demonstrating that pelvic incidence (PI) matches lumbar lordosis (LL) and that increasing pelvic retroversion directly correlates with worsening patient-reported quality-of-life measures. These observations are the cornerstones of contemporary adult spinal deformity surgery and define the goals of reconstructive surgery.

IMAGING

Preoperative evaluation of patients with adult spinal deformity begins with full-length standing 36-in posteroanterior and lateral radiographs (**Fig. 1**). From the lateral image, the physician

A   **B**

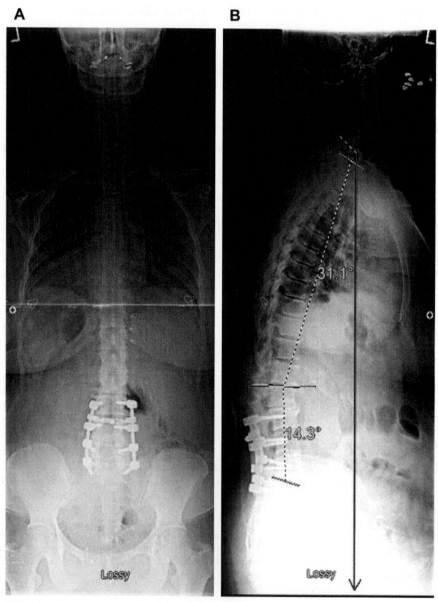

Fig. 1. The 36-in standing posteroanterior (A) and lateral radiographs (B) of a patient with sagittal imbalance.

then measures the patients' LL, PI, sacral slope (SS), pelvic tilt (PT), as well as the sagittal vertical axis (SVA) (**Fig. 2**). The recent introduction of biplanar low-dose radiography (EOS images, EOS Imaging, Inc. Cambridge, MA) allows for improved visualization of the entire spine, skull, and lower extremities[10] (**Fig. 3**); however, this may not be available to all practitioners.

LUMBAR LORDOSIS

LL is defined as the sagittal Cobb angle measurement from the superior end plate of L1 to the sacral end plate (see **Fig. 2**). There is significant variability in what is considered normal LL, and it is more useful to think of the LL as patient specific rather than population based. Specifically, in the well-aligned spine, LL will match PI within 11°. However, as a general rule, between 20° and 70° of LL is considered normal on reaching maturity. Different patterns of lordosis have been reported.[11] Each patient's ideal LL is defined by his or her pelvic

incidence, and a solid understanding of the relationship between PI and LL is essential in the treatment of patients with adult spinal deformity. The amount of segmental lordosis also varies by level, with L4-5 and L5-S1 contributing most of the total lumbar spinal lordosis.

Spondylotic changes, including loss of disk height due to normal aging, generally leads to decreasing lordosis in older patients. LL may also be negatively affected by vertebral compression fractures. One of the most common reasons for symptomatic PI-LL mismatch in contemporary practice is iatrogenic flat back deformity from spinal fusions that are not meticulously planned and performed. This deformity commonly results in a hypolordotic lumbar spine and, when symptomatic, may require corrective surgery.

LL is the sagittal parameter that can be most readily changed with surgery, and reducing a patient's PI-LL mismatch to less than 11° is often a primary goal of adult spinal deformity surgery.[12] LL is a dynamic value; patients' position, supine versus erect, can drastically change this measurement (**Fig. 4**). When planning a deformity correction, a surgeon should evaluate patients' standing, lateral flexion/extension, supine films, and traction radiographs for LL along with either a computed tomography (CT) myelogram or MRI. These images should also be compared with standing radiographs to determine the dynamic component of the patients' deformity. Understanding the flexibility/inflexibility of a specific patient's deformity aids a surgeon in determining which type of surgical deformity technique is most appropriate, for example, anterior lumbar interbody fusion, lateral interbody fusion, transforaminal lumber interbody fusion, or in the case of a rigidly fused spine a pedicle subtraction osteotomy.

PELVIC INCIDENCE

PI is equal to the sum of the PT and SS (PI = SS + PT). Geometrically, this is the angle formed between a line from the center of the femoral head to the midpoint of the sacral end plate and a line orthogonal to the sacral end plate (see **Fig. 2**). PI generally increases during skeletal growth but becomes a fixed, patient-specific quantity at skeletal maturity.[13]

Roussouly and colleagues[14] described how a patients' unique PI influences not only their LL but also their thoracolumbar thoracic and cervical sagittal contours. PI is the foundation on which the spine is built. Because PI is fixed, a loss of LL, either from spondylosis or prior surgery, may result in a mismatch between the PI and LL affecting the patients' global sagittal balance.

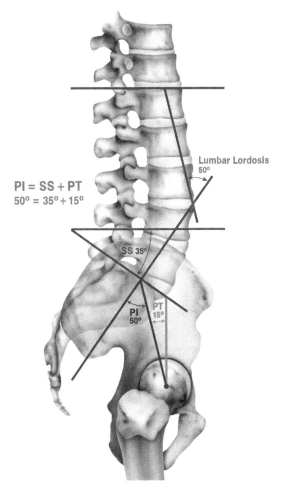

Lumbar Lordosis 50°

$$PI = SS + PT$$
$$50° = 35° + 15°$$

SS 35°

PI 50°   PT 15°

Fig. 2. Line drawing of lumbar spine and pelvis detailing how to measure PI, LL, PT, and SS.

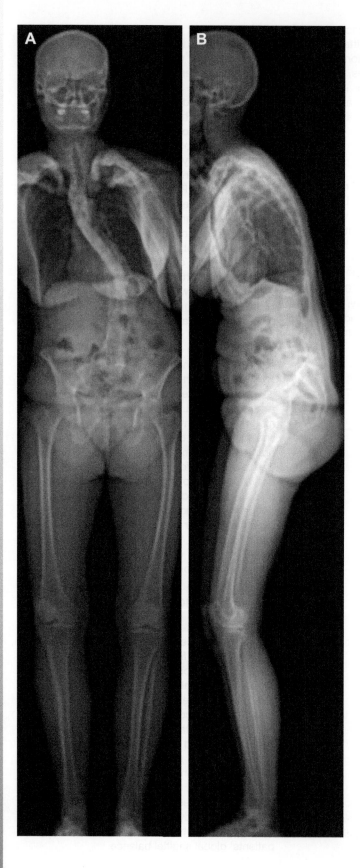

Fig. 3. Standing posteroanterior (*A*) and lateral radiographs (*B*) of a patient with sagittal imbalance taken with an EOS machine.

A   **B**

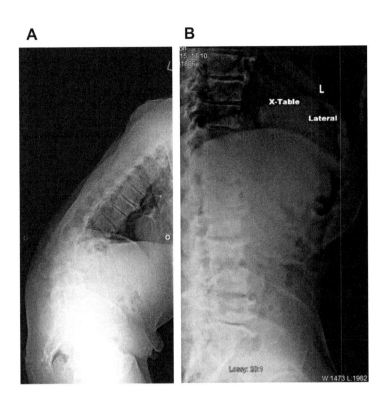

Fig. 4. Standing (*A*) versus supine extension (*B*) lateral radiographs of a patient with sagittal imbalance demonstrating the intrinsic flexibility of the curve.

The work of Schwab and colleagues[15] defines an abnormal LL in relation to PI. The Scoliosis Research Society-Schwab impact-based classification of adult spinal deformity demonstrates a moderate positive correlation between lumbo-pelvic mismatch and disability. Specifically, a PI minus its LL (PI-LL) of greater than 11° is associated with disability based on the Oswestry Disability Index (ODI).[16] Patients with a PI-LL mismatch of greater than 11° have pain with both standing and walking, and a PI-LL difference of greater than 11° is most strongly correlated not only with an ODI greater than 40 but also with an abnormal PT and SVA.[17]

Although PI is a fixed value, its component parts, namely, PT and SS, are not. PI itself can only be changed in skeletally mature patients via sacral osteotomy or pelvic fracture.

PELVIC TILT

PT is the angle formed by a vertical line through the center of the femoral heads and the line from the center of the femoral axis and the midpoint of the sacral end plate (see **Fig. 2**). A normal PT is less than approximately 15°. In response to a loss of LL, patients will increase their PT via hip extension, which is variable and genetically determined, if possible, to achieve normal sagittal balance. Increasing PT is also termed pelvic retroversion. There are limits to the amount of PT that can be

achieved: younger patients may be able to generate more PT as a compensatory mechanism for loss of LL; however, as patients age and begin to lose lumbar flexibility and develop degenerative changes of the hip, their ability to extend through the hips decreases, resulting in sagittal imbalance. Abnormal PT is also easily identified on anterior pelvic radiographs whereby the normal oval appearance of the pelvic outlet narrows as the pelvis PT increases.

An abnormal PT is a compensatory mechanism for spinal deformity, rather than intrinsic to the deformity itself. PT can be thought of as a reservoir to compensate for sagittal balance. Patients are able to compensate for loss of LL and maintain normal sagittal balance by extending through the pelvis. However, there is a limit to this mechanism; when no more PT can be obtained, patients will decompensate and present with global sagittal malalignment.

Surgical intervention does not directly change PT, rather, when patients' LL is brought back into harmony with their PI and this compensatory mechanism is no longer necessary, their PT will improve as the hip reverts from terminal extension and the pelvis rotates forward. It is difficult to plan how much a patient's PT will change with surgery; nevertheless, restoration of PT to less than 25° is a major goal of adult spinal deformity surgery.[12]

An increasing PT directly correlates to increasing symptoms in the setting of adult spinal deformity, and a PT greater than 22° predicts an ODI greater than 40[17]; similarly, increasing PT most directly correlates with pain during ambulation.[9]

SACRAL SLOPE

SS is defined as the angle formed between the horizontal and the sacral end plate (see **Fig. 1**). SS is not a fixed angle, rather it relies on the position of the pelvis relative to the hip axis. SS is inversely correlated with PT; as discussed previously, the sum of the SS and PT is the PI. The lateral radiograph of patients with sagittal imbalance will reveal a horizontal sacrum, increased PT, and loss of LL.

Like PT, lumbar spine surgery indirectly affects SS; however, unlike PT, there is no specific goal for SS restoration. Mathematically, this is because PI is a fixed patient-specific variable and the restoration of the appropriate PT (ie, <25°) is a surgical goal that results in concurrent normalization of the SS. The SS and PT are inversely proportional and equal the PI with all 3 having unique patient-specific values.

WHAT DOES A SURGEON NEED TO KNOW TO PLAN A DEFORMITY CORRECTION?

Although radiographic measurements of spinal deformity, such as PI, LL, and PT, are easy to measure and communicate, they leave out essential information when planning a deformity correction. When evaluating patients with lumbar spinal deformity, a surgeon must *first* take a history. A thorough understanding how pain interferes with activities of daily living versus activities of recreation allows the surgeon to better interpret self-reported scores, such as the ODI and SRS-22r.

Next a surgeon should endeavor to determine the patients' desired outcome from surgery: what can they not do now that they desire to do again? Patients undergoing a lumbar deformity correction who expect to be able to walk a half-mile with minimal pain is reasonable; on the other hand, patients who desire to play competitive tennis at the same level as in their youth may be unrealistic. These nuances are important and can only be elucidated with a thorough history, because all patients will explain that they want to feel better. Only a thorough history allows a surgeon to determine if patients have a realistic expectation of surgery. Often, the authors retake a history, focusing on current symptoms and goals of surgery, at follow-up visits to help provide a more complete understanding of an individual patient's symptoms.

A thorough physical examination is the next step in evaluating patients with spinal deformity. Of all components of the physical examination, watching patients stand and walk is the most important and the most often overlooked. Patients will often be able to compensate for PI-LL mismatch for a short period of time while standing and, thus, will seem to have normal sagittal alignment; on the other hand, these compensatory mechanisms rapidly fail when patients are asked to walk a distance of 50 feet or more. Because the arc of hip flexion and extension is truncated, the patients with loss of sagittal balance and pelvic retroversion will eventually have to lean forward to regain some hip extension to have a more normalized gait pattern. Watching patients walk with and without an assistive device is similarly informative.

After a thorough history and physical examination a surgeon should then carefully evaluate patients' imaging, measuring sagittal imbalance, LL, PI, PT, and SS. The PI-LL mismatch is then calculated. If advanced imaging studies, such as MRI, CT or CT myelogram, are available, they can be used to identify supine LL, along with any concurrent lumbar stenosis, scoliosis, and spondylolisthesis. Alternatively this can be performed via a lateral lumbar spine radiograph with patients supine or over a bolster to evaluate the rigidity of the lumbar spine, which is essential when planning the type of procedure required for a deformity correction.

Now, all the components of lumbar deformity are available to the surgeon and can be interpreted. If a patient with a history of a single level lumbar fusion reports severe pain, but ambulates without sagittal imbalance, has an ODI of 80, no PI-LL mismatch, and a PT of 12°, he or she is not a candidate for a sagittal alignment correction; other sources of pain, such as pseudoarthrosis, should be investigated. However, a patient with a documented solid history of a multilevel lumbar fusion who stands with clinical sagittal imbalance, has an ODI of 50, a PI-LL mismatch of 25°, and 25° PT may be a candidate for lumbar deformity correction. Understanding of and appropriate interpretation of radiographic measures are important guides to deformity correction and an evidence-based approach to the appropriate surgical intervention for patients.

REFERENCES

1. Vasiliadis ES, Grivas TB, Kaspiris A. Historical overview of spinal deformities in ancient Greece. Scoliosis 2009;4:6.
2. Bohler L. The treatment of fractures. Translated from German by Hey Groves EW. 1935.

3. Stagnara P, Mollon G, de Mauroy JC. Reeducation des scolioses. Expansion Scientifique, Paris, France 1978.

4. Duval-Beaupere G, Schmidt C, Cosson P. A barycentremetric study of the sagittal shape of spine and pelvis: the conditions required for an economic standing position. Ann Biomed Eng 1992; 20(4):451–62.

5. Dubousset JCV, Farcy JP, Schwab FJ, et al. Spinal alignment versus spinal balance. St Louis (MO): Quality Medical Publishing; 2015.

6. Duval-Beaupère G, editor. The line of gravity profile view in normal subjects and in anteroposterior spine deformities. Combined Meeting of the Groupe d'Etude de la Scoliose and the Scoliosis Research Society. Montreal, Canada, 1979.

7. Jackson RP, Hales C. Congruent spinopelvic alignment on standing lateral radiographs of adult volunteers. Spine (Phila Pa 1976) 2000;25(21):2808–15.

8. Glassman SD, Berven S, Bridwell K, et al. Correlation of radiographic parameters and clinical symptoms in adult scoliosis. Spine (Phila Pa 1976) 2005; 30(6):682–8.

9. Lafage V, Schwab F, Patel A, et al. Pelvic tilt and truncal inclination: two key radiographic parameters in the setting of adults with spinal deformity. Spine (Phila Pa 1976) 2009;34(17):E599–606.

10. Le Huec JC, Demezon H, Aunoble S. Sagittal parameters of global cervical balance using EOS imaging: normative values from a prospective cohort of asymptomatic volunteers. Eur Spine J 2015; 24(1):63–71.

11. Roussouly P, Nnadi C. Sagittal plane deformity: an overview of interpretation and management. Eur Spine J 2010;19(11):1824–36.

12. Schwab F, Patel A, Ungar B, et al. Adult spinal deformity-postoperative standing imbalance: how much can you tolerate? An overview of key parameters in assessing alignment and planning corrective surgery. Spine (Phila Pa 1976) 2010;35(25):2224–31.

13. Mac-Thiong JM, Berthonnaud E, Dimar JR 2nd, et al. Sagittal alignment of the spine and pelvis during growth. Spine (Phila Pa 1976) 2004;29(15):1642–7.

14. Roussouly P, Gollogly S, Noseda O, et al. The vertical projection of the sum of the ground reactive forces of a standing patient is not the same as the C7 plumb line: a radiographic study of the sagittal alignment of 153 asymptomatic volunteers. Spine (Phila Pa 1976) 2006;31(11):E320–5.

15. Schwab F, Ungar B, Blondel B, et al. Scoliosis Research Society-Schwab adult spinal deformity classification: a validation study. Spine (Phila Pa 1976) 2012;37(12):1077–82.

16. Fairbank JC, Pynsent PB. The Oswestry Disability Index. Spine (Phila Pa 1976) 2000;25(22):2940–52 [discussion: 52].

17. Schwab FJ, Blondel B, Bess S, et al. Radiographical spinopelvic parameters and disability in the setting of adult spinal deformity: a prospective multicenter analysis. Spine (Phila Pa 1976) 2013;38(13):E803–12.

Sagittal Alignment of the Lumbar Spine

Sigurd Berven, MD[a], Rishi Wadhwa, MD[b],*

KEYWORDS

- Sagittal alignment • Adjacent segment degeneration • Lumbo-pelvic mismatch
- Age-adjusted parameters • Surgical planning and strategies

KEY POINTS

- The pathophysiology of lumbar degenerative disease is related to lumbo-pelvic parameters.
- Segmental lordosis is greatest in the L4-5 and L5 to S1 motion segments.
- Normal aging involves progressive forward sagittal alignment and loss of lordosis.
- Restoration of lordosis at L4 to S1 is a priority for lumbar spine reconstructive procedures.
- Inadequate restoration of lordosis at L4 to S1 is an important factor in adjacent segment degeneration.

INTRODUCTION

Sagittal alignment of the lumbar spine has an important and measurable impact on the pathogenesis of lumbar spine disorders and on health-related quality of life in pediatric and adult populations. Lordosis in the lumbar spine is a unique feature of the human spine and fundamental to the development of an upright, bipedal posture and gait.[1] Understanding lumbar lordosis and the relationship between lumbar lordosis, pelvic incidence, and balance or alignment of the spine is essential for the study of pathogenesis of lumbar developmental and degenerative conditions and for informed planning for spinal reconstruction. Sagittal alignment in the lumbar spine includes consideration of the sagittal Cobb angle, or lumbar lordosis, as well as lumbo-pelvic parameters, including the relationship of lumbar lordosis to pelvic incidence, and the tilt of the pelvis. Sagittal alignment in the lumbar spine changes with age and with degenerative pathologies. The appropriate alignment of the lumbar spine and the goals for realignment procedures are different in adolescents and young adults compared with elderly patients. The purpose of this article is to define normal lumbar lordosis and lumbo-pelvic parameters, to discuss the relationship between lumbar alignment and lumbo-pelvic balance with the pathogenesis of lumbar degenerative pathologies, and to guide an evidence-based approach to surgical planning for realignment of the lumbar spine.

MEASURING SAGITTAL ALIGNMENT IN THE LUMBAR SPINE

Understanding normal alignment of the lumbar spine is fundamental to the study of lumbar developmental and degenerative pathologies and is a prerequisite for an evidence-based approach to surgical planning for reconstructive procedures. The sagittal alignment of the normal lumbar spine is lordotic, and the amount of lordosis varies significantly between normal adults. Lumbar lordosis is conventionally measured from the upper end plate of T12 to the upper end plate of the sacrum. There is significant variability in lumbar lordosis between

Disclosure Statement: The authors have nothing to disclose.
[a] Orthopedic Surgery, UCSF Spine Center, 400 Parnassus Avenue, San Francisco, CA 94143, USA;
[b] Neurosurgery, UCSF Spine Center, 400 Parnassus Avenue, San Francisco, CA 94143, USA
* Corresponding author. 1100 South Eliseo Drive, Suite 1, Greenbrae, CA 94904.
E-mail address: Rishi.wadhwa@ucsf.edu

Neurosurg Clin N Am 29 (2018) 331–339
https://doi.org/10.1016/j.nec.2018.03.009

normal, asymptomatic adults. Bernhardt and Bridwell[2] studied the normal segmental alignment of the thoracic and lumbar spine in order to provide a guide for the goals of realignment procedures. The investigators identified significant variability in the absolute lordosis between individuals; but they recognized a clear pattern of increase in lumbar lordosis from the upper to the lower lumbar segments, with two-thirds of the lumbar lordosis occurring from the L4 to S1 segments. The observation that most lordosis is in the lower 2 segments of the lumbar region is an important observation regarding appropriate procedures for lumbar spine reconstruction and supports a strategy for realignment of the lower lumbar spine with restoration of segmental lordosis to equal two-thirds of the total lordotic goal. The emphasis on the lower lumbar spine in realignment procedures is especially important because many lumbar degenerative and developmental pathologies involve the lower lumbar spine and lumbosacral region of the spine.

Dubousset[3] identified the importance of the pelvic vertebra in sagittal alignment of the spine. Specifically, in his great breakthrough in understanding 3-dimensional alignment of the spine, Dubousset[3] recognized that the sagittal alignment of the spine involves a linked succession of balanced curves from the head to the pelvis. He cites the work of Duval-Beaupere in defining the fundamental importance of the "incidence angle" or pelvic incidence in defining the lumbar lordosis in a balanced or aligned spine. In order to maintain a balanced standing upright posture with minimal energy expenditure, an optimal alignment of the lumbar spine is determined by the intrinsic alignment or incidence of the pelvis. In reconstructive surgery for patients with spinal deformity, Dubousset[3] recognized that balance, alignment, and motion of the spine are determined by lumbo-pelvic alignment and pelvic compensation for sagittal alignment in the thoracic and lumbar spine. Therefore, spinal balance, or alignment, depends on a match of lumbar lordosis and pelvic incidence. With this background, we may understand the impact of lumbo-pelvic parameters and mismatches on the pathogenesis of lumbar developmental and degenerative conditions and on health status.

LUMBO-PELVIC PARAMETERS AND THE PATHOGENESIS OF DEGENERATIVE AND DEVELOPMENTAL PATHOLOGIES IN THE LUMBAR SPINE

Lumbo-pelvic parameters have an important and measurable impact on the pathogenesis of lumbar developmental and degenerative pathology and on the impact of spinal deformity on health-related quality of life. Rousouly and colleagues[4] described the variants of normal sagittal alignment in the lumbar spine and pelvis and postulated correlations between alignment and lumbar degenerative and developmental pathologies. The investigators identified 4 specific variants sagittal alignment defined by the apex of the thoracic and lumbar curves, the inflection point between the thoracic and lumbar curve, the sacral slope, the total kyphosis and lordosis of the thoracic and lumbar spine, and the arc of lordosis of the upper and lower lumbar spine. The arc of the lower lumbar spine is most variable, and highly correlated with sacral slope. Patients with a lower lumbar lordosis and a more horizontal sacrum (type 1 and 2) are more likely to develop lumbar degenerative pathologies including symptomatic lumbar disc degeneration and disc herniation. Patients with a higher sacral slope and correlating pelvic incidence and a higher apex of lordosis (L3 or above) are more likely to develop symptoms of spinal stenosis. The correlation between lumbar lordosis, sacral slope, and location of lordosis and lumbar degenerative pathologies demonstrates an important causative relationship in the pathogenesis of lumbar degenerative disorders.[5-8] Roussouly and colleagues[9] conclude that restoration of lumbar lordosis in the lower lumbar spine is biomechanically a priority, especially in patients with a higher pelvic incidence.

The relationship between lumbo-pelvic parameters and the development of spondylolisthesis has been well established. Biomechanically, patients with a high pelvic incidence have high sacral slope and an anterior displacement of their center axis of gravity relative to the posterior elements of the sacrum, resulting in high shear forces across the lumbosacral junction. Labelle and colleagues[10,11] demonstrated that spinopelvic balance is an important factor in the pathogenesis of developmental spondylolisthesis. Specifically, patients with a high sacral slope and high pelvic incidence are likely to develop developmental listhesis, whereas patients with a low sacral slope and low pelvic incidence are likely to develop acquired olisthesis. Mac-Thiong and Labelle[12] proposed a classification of spondylolisthesis that is based on spinopelvic parameters and global alignment of the spine. The classification has a strong correlation with the health status of patients and supports a surgical strategy that involves more invasive approaches to reduce spinopelvic malalignment and global sagittal alignment in patients with more severe deformity.

In adult spinal deformity, lumbo-pelvic parameters are a significant determinant of health status; restoration of lumbo-pelvic alignment is an important goal of surgical management of deformity. In work to define the radiographic parameters that determine the health status of patients with symptomatic adult spinal deformity, Schwab and colleagues[13] initially identified lumbar lordosis as an important predictor of disability and a determinant of clinical impact. However, subsequent work demonstrated that lumbar lordosis alone was a less significant predictor of clinical impact of deformity than lumbo-pelvic parameters, including the relationship between lumbar lordosis and pelvic incidence and the pelvic tilt.[14] The high correlation between radiographic parameters of global sagittal alignment of the spine, pelvic tilt, and match of lumbar lordosis and pelvic incidence with health-related quality of life provide the basis for restoration of those parameters as the central goal of reconstructive surgery in the adult with spinal deformity. It is important to recognize that in elderly patients, normal global sagittal alignment is significantly anterior compared with adolescents and young adults and lumbar lordosis is significantly less. Gelb and colleagues[15] demonstrated that global alignment of the spine may be up to 8 cm anterior to the posterior margin of the sacrum in asymptomatic patients older than 60 years. Therefore, adjustment of sagittal alignment goals in elderly patients may include a higher sagittal vertical axis and a higher mismatch between lordosis and pelvic incidence.[16,17]

The relationship between lumbo-pelvic parameters and adjacent segment degeneration is a strong correlation and has important implications regarding appropriate management of lumbar degenerative pathology. Kumar and colleagues[18] demonstrated that patients who were fused with a positive global sagittal alignment and a vertical sacrum were significantly more likely to develop adjacent segment degeneration requiring revision surgery within 5 years.

In adult deformity surgery, patients with an inharmonious global lumbar lordosis and a greater lordosis in the upper lumbar spine compared with the lower lumbar spine are more likely to develop thoracolumbar junctional failure.[19] In lumbar degenerative pathology, an inadequate restoration of lordosis in the region of L4 to S1 is a strong risk factor for adjacent segment degeneration. Biomechanically, the shear forces at the adjacent segment are significantly higher in patients who have an inadequate restoration of lordosis in the lower lumbar spine compared with pelvic incidence.[20] Senteler and colleagues[20] demonstrated higher shear forces at the L3-4 intervertebral level after L4 to S1 fusion

Table 1
Summary of selected references

Author	Contribution
Chopin	Patients fused in a positive global sagittal alignment and with a vertical sacrum were more likely to develop adjacent segment disease requiring revision surgery.
Dubousset	Recognized the sagittal alignment of the spine involves a linked succession of balanced curves from the head to the pelvis.
Roussouly	Restoration of lumbar lordosis in the lower lumbar spine is biomechanically a priority, especially in patients with a higher pelvic incidence.
Gelb	In the elderly, sagittal alignment may be up to 8 cm positive in asymptomatic patients older than 60 y.
Senteler	Higher shear forces were demonstrated at L3-4 in patients after L4 to S1 fusion whose LL-PI was mismatched (inadequate restoration).

Abbreviation: LL-PI, lumbar lordosis–pelvic incidence.

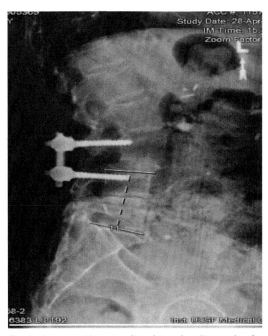

Fig. 1. Preoperative standing lateral radiograph of a 56-year-old man with prior fusion at L3-4 and symptomatic degenerative changes at L4 to S1. Patient is hypolordotic at L3 to S1 with compensatory hyperlordosis at L1 to L3.

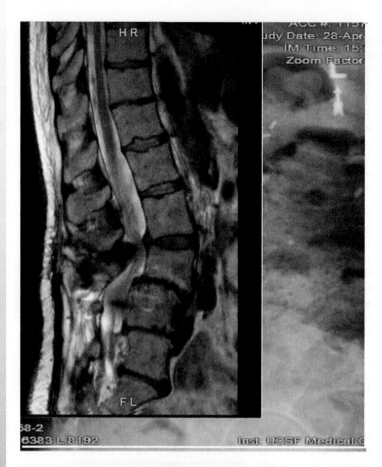

Fig. 2. Preoperative MRI demonstrates severe stenosis adjacent to the hypolordotic L3 to S1 segments. There is limited mobility at the L4 to S1 segments in the supine posture.

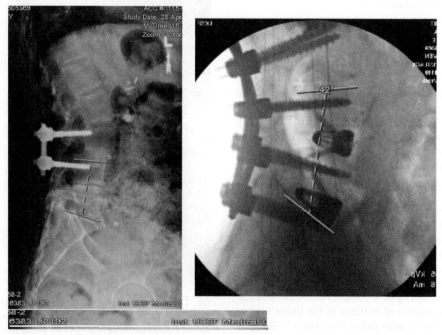

Fig. 3. Restoration of lordosis from L4 to S1 with anterior column reconstruction using hyperlordotic anterior lumbar interbody fusions at L4 to S1 and TLIF at L2-3.

by changing segmental motion constraints thereby leading to an increased chance of disk degeneration. They described an approximate linear relationship between sagittal alignment and intervertebral loads, in addition describing higher shear forces at L3-4 in patients who are clinically observed to be prone to adjacent segment disease. These shear forces at L3-4 were higher in L4-5 fusion and even more so significantly in patients with L4 to S1 fusion. Their conclusion was to maximize lordosis in hypolordotic patients at L4 to S1 to minimize shear stresses at L3-4. They also suggested that shear forces differed to a larger degree than compression forces in different alignments after fusion, in agreement with other articles demonstrating that shear forces were more responsible for creating degenerative forces at adjacent levels as opposed to compressive forces. The clinical association between inadequate restoration of lumbar lordosis in the lower lumbar spine and adjacent segment degeneration is high, and spinopelvic malalignment is the primary risk factor for adjacent segment degeneration in reconstructive surgery for lumbar degenerative pathology.[21,22] In degenerative pathology and spinal deformity, the goal of restoring lumbar lordosis, especially in the region of L4 to S1, is an important priority to avoid symptomatic adjacent segment degeneration. **Table 1** provides a summary for the key references cited.

PREOPERATIVE PLANNING
Preoperative Planning

Measurements and examination
It is important to think of spine surgery, even for 1 or 2 levels, in a global sense. Preservation and restoration of sagittal alignment is paramount to prevent flat-back syndrome. Physical examination should include evaluating for pelvic obliquity, stooped forward posture with knee flexion, as well as the relation of the head to the pelvis. If possible, 36-in standing radiographs should be obtained in all patients. Pelvic parameters should be measured to compare lumbar lordosis and pelvic incidence and what corrective measures should be performed to accomplish lumbar lordosis–pelvic incidence match within 10°. The sagittal vertical axis should be within 5 to 6 cm from the posterior margin of the sacrum. Patients should be examined to see if any deformity is reducible with positioning versus a fixed deformity, which will not reduce with physical examination manipulation.

Continuum of correction
Preoperative planning gives an adequate estimate of what goals should be achieved in surgery with

an understanding that corrective measurements exist on a continuum. For instance, a grade 3 osteotomy (pedicle subtraction osteotomy) can be accomplished more easily after performing the necessary steps for a grade 2 osteotomy (Smith-Petersen osteotomy). If one keeps in mind the principles of osteotomies, one corrective measure naturally leads to the next in a continuum.

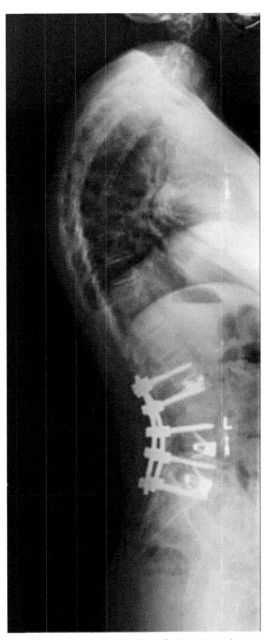

Fig. 4. Standing lateral view of the spine demonstrating restoration of a matched lumbar lordosis and pelvic incidence, with restoration of lordosis primarily at L4 to S1.

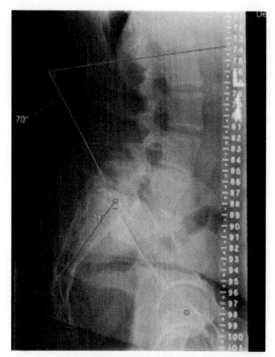

Fig. 5. Lateral radiograph demonstrating lumbar spondylolisthesis and pelvic parameters.

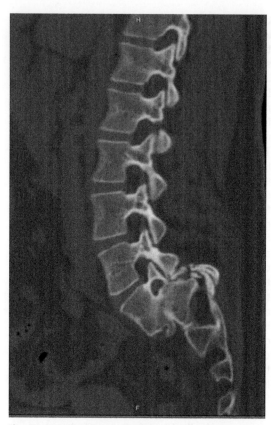

Fig. 7. Computed tomography scan showing osseous fusion of the spondylolisthesis.

Preoperative health status

It is of utmost importance to understand patients' preoperative health status before the operation. Even though patients may benefit from a larger correction, they may not be able to tolerate the surgery secondary to existing morbidities. In these instances, it is important to remember to treat the patients and not the images. The surgical plan can be tailored to get patients relief while minimizing complications. Risk stratification can be completed before the operation to carefully select patients for operations and to ensure success.

Reestablishing lordosis at L4-5, L5 to S1

Most lordosis in the lumbar spine naturally occurs at L4-5 and L5 to S1. It is important to restore lordosis at these levels. Minimizing shear forces at the mid and upper lumbar spine can be accomplished by achieving lordosis at the lower levels. Ultimately the goal is to minimize proximal failure, adjacent level disease, as well as improper correction of the spine.

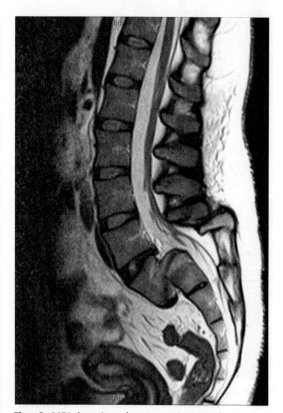

Fig. 6. MRI imaging demonstrating grade 3 to 4 spondylolisthesis.

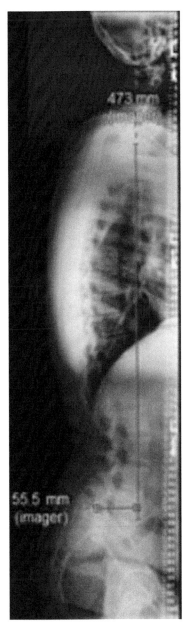

Fig. 8. The 36-in standing radiographs showing preserved sagittal balance.

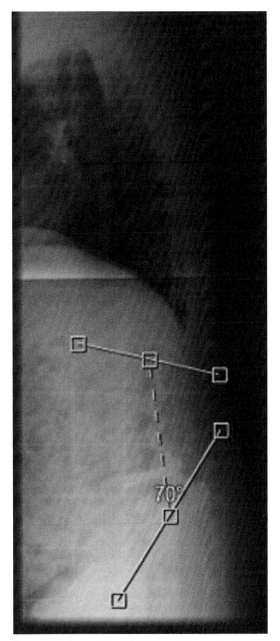

Fig. 9. Postoperative lateral radiograph demonstrating preserved pelvic parameters.

Case 1 A 56-year-old man was treated with a posterolateral fusion at L3-4 for spondylolisthesis (Fig. 1). This patient presented with symptomatic adjacent segment degeneration and stenosis at L2-3 and advanced degenerative changes at L4 to S1 (Fig. 2). Revision surgery involved an anterior spine fusion from L4 to S1 to restore lumbar lordosis to the lower lumbar spine and decompression and transforaminal lumbar interbody fusion (TLIF) at L2-3 for adjacent segment stenosis (Figs. 3 and 4).

Case 2 A 32-year-old woman presented with chronic back pain, which had worsened over the past few years. She also presented with bilateral L5 radiculopathy. Imaging showed evidence of grade 3 to 4 lumbar spondylolisthesis (Fig. 5). Dynamic imaging showed no gross instability, and MRI showed tethered bilateral L5 roots (Fig. 6) and L5 to S1 osseous fusion (Fig. 7). Preoperative pelvic parameters showed a preoperative lumbar lordosis/pelvic incidence agreement (<10°) (see

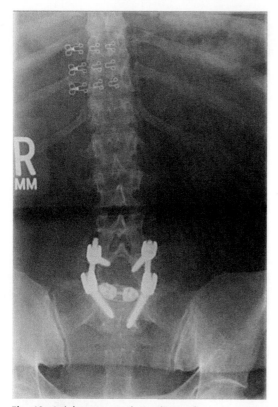

Fig. 10. Axial postoperative radiograph.

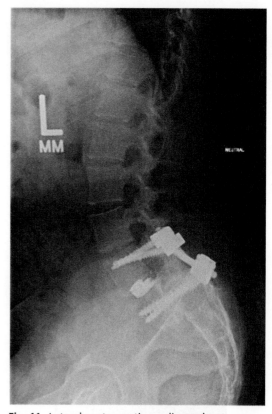

Fig. 11. Lateral postoperative radiograph.

Fig. 5). Sagittal alignment (Fig. 8) was within normal limits as well; the authors took great care to preserve her parameters and to not over-correct her, as that could lead to pseudoarthrosis, sacral insufficiency fracture, and/or screw failure/pullout.

She underwent L4 to S1 fusion with an L4-5 TLIF and L5 to S1 transosseous screw and L5

pedicle resection for decompression. She toler-ated the procedure well, and the authors were able to preserve her alignment and not undercorrect/overcorrect her spine (Fig. 9). Her lumbo-pelvic parameters were similar to the pre-operative parameters. She is doing well at 2 years' follow-up with solid arthrodesis (see Fig. 9; Figs. 10–12).

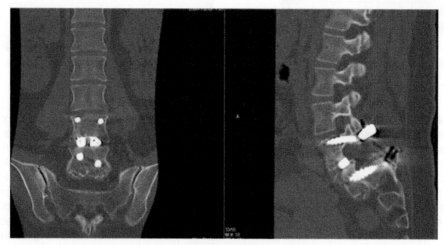

Fig. 12. Computed tomography scan demonstrating successful L4 to S1 fusion.

SUMMARY

Lordosis in the lumbar spine is a uniquely human feature that permits upright, bipedal stance with economy of energy expenditure. There is significant variability of lordosis in normal, asymptomatic spines; appropriate lordosis is determined by pelvic incidence and influenced by age and degenerative pathology. The relationship of lumbar lordosis and pelvic incidence is an important determinant of the pathophysiology of lumbar developmental and degenerative pathology. In reconstructing the spine affected by degenerative pathology or deformity, goals of realignment must prioritize restoration of lumbo-pelvic parameters. Most lumbar lordosis occurs from L4 to S1, and restoration of lordosis in the lower lumbar spine is especially important to avoid junctional failure and adjacent segment degeneration.

REFERENCES

1. Berge C. Heterochronic processes in human evolution: an ontogenetic analysis of the hominid pelvis. Am J Phys Anthropol 1998;105(4):441–59.
2. Bernhardt M, Bridwell KH. Segmental analysis of the sagittal plane alignment of the normal thoracic and lumbar spines and thoracolumbar junction. Spine 1989;14(7):717–21.
3. Dubousset J. Three-dimensional analysis of the scoliotic deformity. In: Weinstein SL, editor. The pediatric spine: principles and practice. New York: Raven Press; 1994. p. 479–96.
4. Roussouly P, Gollogly S, Berthonnaud E, et al. Classification of the normal variation in the sagittal alignment of the human lumbar spine and pelvis in the standing position. Spine (Phila Pa 1976) 2005;30(3):346–53.
5. Jackson RP, McManus AC. Radiographic analysis of sagittal plane alignment and balance in standing volunteers and patients with low back pain matched for age, sex, and size: a prospective controlled clinical study. Spine 1994;19:1611–8.
6. Evcik D, Yucel A. Lumbar lordosis in acute and chronic low back pain patients. Rheumatol Int 2003;23:163–5.
7. Barrey C, Jund J, Noseda O, et al. Sagittal balance of the pelvis-spine complex and lumbar degenerative diseases. A comparative study about 85 cases. Eur Spine J 2007;16(9):1459–67.
8. Chaléat-Valayer E, Mac-Thiong JM, Paquet J, et al. Sagittal spino-pelvic alignment in chronic low back pain. Eur Spine J 2011;20(Suppl 5):634–40.
9. Roussouly P, Pinheiro-Franco JL. Biomechanical analysis of the spino-pelvic organization and adaptation in pathology. Eur Spine J 2011;20(Suppl 5):609–18.
10. Labelle H, Roussouly P, Berthonnaud E, et al. Developmental spondylolisthesis: the importance of spino-pelvic balance in L5-s1 developmental spondylolisthesis: a review of pertinent radiologic measurements [review]. Spine (Phila Pa 1976) 2005;30(6 Suppl):S27–34.
11. Labelle H, Roussouly P, Berthonnaud E, et al. Spondylolisthesis, pelvic incidence, and spinopelvic balance: a correlation study. Spine (Phila Pa 1976) 2004;29(18):2049 54.
12. Mac-Thiong JM, Labelle H. A proposal for a surgical classification of pediatric lumbosacral spondylolisthesis based on current literature. Eur Spine J 2006;15(10):1425–35.
13. Schwab F, Farcy JP, Bridwell K, et al. A clinical impact classification of scoliosis in the adult. Spine 2006;31(18):2109–14.
14. Schwab F, Farcy JP, Bridwell K, et al, International Spine Study Group. The SRS-Schwab adult spinal deformity classification: assessment and clinical correlations based on a prospective operative and nonoperative cohort. Neurosurgery 2013;73(4):559–68.
15. Gelb DE, Lenke LG, Bridwell KH, et al. An analysis of sagittal spinal alignment in 100 asymptomatic middle and older aged volunteers. Spine (Phila Pa 1976) 1995;20(12):1351–8.
16. Lafage R, Schwab F, Glassman S, et al, International Spine Study Group. Age-adjusted alignment goals have the potential to reduce PJK. Spine (Phila Pa 1976) 2017;42(17):1275–82.
17. Lafage R, Schwab F, Challier V, et al, International Spine Study Group. Defining spino-pelvic alignment thresholds: should operative goals in adult spinal deformity surgery account for age? Spine (Phila Pa 1976) 2016;41(1):62–8.
18. Kumar MN, Baklanov A, Chopin D. Correlation between sagittal plane changes and adjacent segment degeneration following lumbar spine fusion. Eur Spine J 2001;10:314–9.
19. Faundez AA, Richards J, Maxy P, et al. The mechanism in junctional failure of thoraco-lumbar fusions. Part II: analysis of a series of PJK after thoracolumbar fusion to determine parameters allowing to predict the risk of junctional breakdown. Eur Spine J 2018;27(Suppl 1):139–48.
20. Senteler M, Weisse B, Snedeker JG, et al. Pelvic incidence-lumbar lordosis mismatch results in increased segmental joint loads in the unfused and fused lumbar spine. Eur Spine J 2014;23(7):1384–93.
21. Rothenfluh DA, Mueller DA, Rothenfluh E, et al. Pelvic incidence-lumbar lordosis mismatch predisposes to adjacent segment disease after lumbar spinal fusion. Eur Spine J 2015;24(6):1251–8.
22. Di Martino A, Quattrocchi CC, Scarciolla L, et al. Estimating the risk for symptomatic adjacent segment degeneration after lumbar fusion: analysis from a cohort of patients undergoing revision surgery. Eur Spine J 2014;23(Suppl 6):693–8.

Approach Selection
Multiple Anterior Lumbar Interbody Fusion to Recreate Lumbar Lordosis Versus Pedicle Subtraction Osteotomy: When, Why, How?

Andrew K. Chan, MD[a],*, Praveen V. Mummaneni, MD[a],
Christopher I. Shaffrey, MD[b]

KEYWORDS

- Anterior lumbar interbody fusion • Pedicle subtraction osteotomy • Lumbar lordosis
- Sagittal imbalance

KEY POINTS

- Multilevel ALIFs or PSO may be used to achieve restoration of lumbar lordosis and correct sagittal alignment in well-selected patients.
- Potential advantages of the multilevel ALIF technique include lower morbidity, blood loss, and decreased risk of neurologic complications at the cost of approach-specific complications including retrograde ejaculation and vascular and visceral injury.
- Potential advantages of the PSO technique include a generally greater single-level lordotic correction, the ability to correct multiplanar deformity when done asymmetrically, and avoidance of anterior scarring and adhesions in patients with a prior history of anterior spinal or abdominal surgery.
- Disadvantages of PSO include a higher complication rate, blood loss, and a more technically demanding procedure.

INTRODUCTION

In adult spinal deformity (ASD), the loss of lumbar lordosis (LL) leads to a series of compensatory spinopelvic changes to maintain global spinal balance. Ultimately these mechanisms may fail, leading to sagittal malalignment, functional impairment, disability, and impaired quality of life.[1–3] There are multiple causes for the loss of LL, including lumbar degenerative disease, post-laminectomy kyphosis, post-traumatic kyphosis, iatrogenic flat back syndrome, and ankylosing spondylitis.[4–6] In the case of iatrogenic flat back syndrome, inadequately restoring LL is associated with the development of adjacent segment degeneration.[7,8] For well-selected patients who fail conservative management strategies, spinal deformity surgery is indicated. The surgical goal of deformity surgery in the adult includes restoration of lumbar alignment in the sagittal and coronal planes.

Disclosure Statement: Dr P.V. Mummaneni is a consultant for DePuy Spine and Stryker and has direct stock ownership in Spinicity/ISD. He receives royalties from DePuy Spine, Thieme Publishers, and Springer Publishers. He has received honoraria from Globus. Dr C.I. Shaffrey has direct stock ownership in, is a consultant for, and a patent holder with NuVasive. He is a consultant and patent holder for Zimmer Biomet. He is a patent holder with Medtronic.
[a] Department of Neurological Surgery, University of California, San Francisco, 505 Parnassus Avenue M779, San Francisco, CA 94143, USA; [b] Department of Neurosurgery, University of Virginia, PO Box 800386, Charlottesville, VA 22908, USA
* Corresponding author.
E-mail address: Andrew.chan@ucsf.edu

Neurosurg Clin N Am 29 (2018) 341–354
https://doi.org/10.1016/j.nec.2018.03.004
1042-3680/18/

In addition to correction of sagittal vertical axis (SVA) and pelvic tilt (PT), restoration of physiologic LL is a fundamental principle of spinal deformity surgery and portends better long-term outcomes.[2,3,9–12] For a given pelvic incidence (PI), restoration of LL that is within $10°$ of PI is considered optimal.[13] Thus, the magnitude of correction necessary for LL is directly proportional to the magnitude of preoperative PI-LL mismatch for a given patient. Patients that are able to achieve an optimization of PI-LL mismatch have been shown to have superior outcomes following spinal deformity surgery.[4,12,14]

Both anterior and posterior-based approaches have been described to correct lumbar hypolordosis and each hold unique advantages and disadvantages. This article discusses the indications, techniques, and complications for an anterior-based approach (multilevel anterior lumbar interbody fusion [ALIF]) and a posterior-based approach (pedicle subtraction osteotomy [PSO]).

MULTILEVEL ANTERIOR LUMBAR INTERBODY FUSION

The ALIF technique permits segmental realignment of the lumbar spine through the intervertebral disk. The technique is appropriate for multiple causes of lumbar degenerative deformity including degenerative scoliosis, postlaminectomy deformity, and adjacent segment degeneration. The primary prerequisite for ALIF is an intervertebral disk space through which the surgeon may gain segmental realignment of the spine. The ALIF approach permits complete release of the anterior longitudinal ligament and annulus fibrosis, facilitating lordotic correction. A primary advantage of the anterior approach lies in its avoidance of the invasiveness of the posterior approach. In the case of the multilevel ALIF, the approach altogether avoids risk to the neural structures and significant manipulation of posterior musculature, depending on the posterior instrumentation technique (eg, minimally invasive, percutaneous). The multilevel ALIF accomplishes the goal of lordotic correction without compromising the posterior tension band. Additionally, it avoids the significant morbidity and high blood loss associated with three-column osteotomies, such as PSO.

Biomechanically, the multilevel ALIF offers several advantages. The multilevel ALIF more harmoniously imitates the natural gradual segmental LL of the spine.[15] This is contrasted by the abrupt angular correction at the index level of PSO. Biomechanical studies suggest that ALIF may limit the destabilization of axial

rotational stability seen with lumbar PSO[16]; this potentially decreases the mechanical demand on posterior instrumentation and may limit rod fractures, hardware failure, and pseudarthrosis. Circumferential fusion of the lumbosacral junction is especially useful to avoid pseudarthrosis and implant failure.

A disadvantage is that the multilevel ALIF may require an additional posterior approach to facilitate spinal realignment with posterior-based mobilization of the spine, to reduce loss of correction, and to prevent pseudarthrosis or interbody cage subsidence. Posterior fixation may be accomplished by either a one-stage, two-approach procedure or a two-stage procedure, both of which may potentially lead to increased anesthesia time.

In a comparison with posterior-only surgeries for ASD, the combined ALIF and Posterior Spinal Fusion (PSF) approach has been shown to achieve largely equivalent results with significant improvements in health-related quality of life measures and radiographic outcomes, including LL.[17] Furthermore, in a study of 42 patients who underwent the multilevel ALIF for restoration of LL, excellent LL and PI matching was accomplished, with an average LL correction of nearly $30°$ at 2-year follow-up.[18] This is similar to the 30-degree correction associated with a PSO.

Indications

The multilevel ALIF is appropriate for patients who have moderate-to-severe sagittal deformity who require a gradual correction in LL across several segments. The patient with a loss of lordosis on standing films with mobility on flexion/extension views, or on supine radiograph or computed tomography may be most appropriate for a multilevel anterior lumbar approach to the spine. Patients with loss of lordosis over the segments of L4 to S1 are appropriate for ALIF reconstruction to restore the appropriate alignment of the lower lumbar spine. It is less appropriate for those who require a larger angular correction at a single level in conditions including congenital kyphosis or post-traumatic deformity, for which the posterior-based PSO may be better suited. **Table 1** outlines the indications for multilevel ALIF and for PSO in the restoration of LL.

The multilevel ALIF is also advantageous in several unique clinical situations. The multilevel ALIF is generally a lower morbidity procedure than the three-column PSO in cases where a solid anterior column fusion is not present. The multilevel ALIF usually has substantially less blood loss than PSO procedures and may be preferred in more frail

Table 1
Indications for multilevel ALIF and PSO in the treatment of flat back deformity

Multilevel ALIF	PSO
Moderate-to-severe sagittal deformity	Moderate-to-severe sagittal deformity
Does not require a large angular correction at a single level	Require a large angular correction at a single level
Patients who are less tolerant of medical or surgical complications (eg, frail, elderly, presence of significant comorbidity) and intraoperative blood loss	Patients who can tolerate the high risk of medical or surgical complications and intraoperative blood loss
In patients with prior posterior spinal fusion in which the surgeon wishes to avoid the complex exposure and dissection of scar	In patients with a prior anterior abdominal/spinal surgical history
Availability of spinal surgeon with expertise in the anterior approach to the spine or vascular approach surgeon	Lack of experience with anterior approach to the spine or unavailability of vascular approach surgeon
In patients also requiring: • Restoration of disk space height • Indirect nerve root decompression • Release of anterior longitudinal ligament • A wide discectomy • Insertion of large, wedge-shaped lordotic grafts	In patients also requiring: • Simultaneous multiplanar correction (asymmetric PSO) • An open posterior approach for concomitant pathology (multilevel spinal stenosis requiring decompression) • Maintenance of fertility (retrograde ejaculation risk with ALIF) • One-stage revision surgery following a posterior fusion (multilevel ALIF lordotic correction may be limited by dorsal hardware)

patients, elderly patients, or those with significant medical comorbidities. However, the multilevel ALIF is generally contraindicated in patients with extensive artherosclerotic vascular calcification, prior retroperitoneal surgery, or irradiation.

In patients with concomitant foraminal stenosis and radiculopathy, the anterior-based multilevel ALIF can provide indirect decompression of the nerve root foramen at each level via a restoration of disk space height. The anterior approach facilitates a wide release of the disk space by removal of the anterior longitudinal ligament and annulus fibrosis and the ability to remove all of the nucleus pulposis. The large opening simplifies placement of large footprint interbody devices that resist subsidence. The circumferential disk space release coupled with higher-angled (hyperlordotic) design facilitates segmental correction enhancing restoration of LL.

In patients with prior posterior spinal surgery, an advantage of multilevel ALIF is that it avoids the complexity and morbidity associated with dissection of the previous surgical scar needed for a PSO. However, in the case of iatrogenic flatback deformity caused by prior lumbar instrumentation, the multilevel ALIF approach may require a 3-stage back-front-back approach, wherein the posterior instrumentation is removed before anterior multilevel ALIF correction and subsequent posterior reinstrumentation. This also adds to the surgical complexity, operative length, and may require repeated patient positioning and a staged surgery. Some prefer PSO in this scenario because the removal of previous instrumentation and lordotic correction is achieved with a single approach. Recent preliminary studies demonstrate the feasibility of using hyperlordotic cages anteriorly (without prior removal of posterior instrumentation) to "overpower" posterior instrumentation, allowing for anterior lordotic correction without a back-front-back approach.[19,20] This front-back approach may be well suited to managing flat back in the setting of lumbar pseudarthrosis resulting from a posterior spinal fusion.

Ultimately, surgeon preference and availability of a specialized approach general or vascular surgeon may determine the ability to proceed with the multilevel ALIF approach.

Technique

Level selection and correction planning
The amount of segmental LL correction should be determined to optimize PI-LL mismatch within 10°.

Additionally, approximately two-thirds of physiologic LL arises from the L4-S1 levels. Anterior interbody correction should aim to restore these physiologic relationships. Interbody devices should be chosen with sufficient lordotic angle to achieve this goal. This usually requires placement of an interbody device with more lordosis than planning indicates unless subsequent posterior column osteotomies are planned. Generally, interbody devices cannot be placed higher than L2-3 using an anterior paramedian approach, and a direct lateral or prepsoas approach may be most useful for anterior interbody release and fusion above L2. **Fig. 1** demonstrates preoperative and postoperative lateral radiographs of a patient who underwent multilevel ALIF to restore LL (preoperative LL 44°, postoperative LL 60°). This was accomplished with a three-level (L3-4, L4-5, L5-S1) multilevel ALIF.

Surgical technique

To minimize complications, the multilevel ALIF should be performed with either a surgeon experienced with the anterior approach (and handling the complications) or with an approach surgeon. In multiple studies, surgeries performed with a combined vascular and spine surgery team were associated with a lower rate of vascular injury and a shorter operative time.[21,22]

If a multilevel ALIF is planned, the surgeon should consider obtaining preoperative angiographic imaging (computed tomography or magnetic resonance with angiography) assessing for any atypical vascular anatomy. This is especially important for higher-level ALIF levels, where an aberrant lower pole renal artery may be present and encountered at L2-3 or L3-4 levels (~5% of patients[22]). Access to the anterior lumbar spine involves mobilization of iliac arteries and veins and thus obtaining detailed preoperative imaging helps to prevent unintended vascular injury. For example, in patients with severe arthrosclerosis, arterial elasticity is diminished limiting the degree of safe retraction and exposure to the anterior disk space. Although most cases ultimately involve minimal blood loss, it is important to prepare for catastrophic blood loss should vascular injury occur. Adequate intravenous and arterial access should be established and intraoperative cell saver may be used.

The patient is positioned supine with the surgeons standing to the side of the patient. The patient may be hyperextended with a small bump (eg, intravenous bag) placed under the lumbosacral junction, or extension of the table across the lumbosacral region of the spine. Pressure points are padded appropriately. C-arm fluoroscopy facilitates incision planning.

Generally, a left-sided retroperitoneal approach is performed. However, in those who have a history of prior abdominal, gynecologic, genitourinary, or anterior spinal surgery, or those in which further anterior surgery is anticipated, a right-sided retroperitoneal approach or transperitoneal approach may be used.[23]

A left paramedian vertical incision is performed. Muscular paralysis aids the exposure. A longitudinal incision of the anterior rectus sheath is performed. The rectus muscle is then reflected laterally. Below the arcuate line, the posterior rectus sheath and the transversalis fascia is divided.

Dissection continues until the peritoneum is identified. The retroperitoneum is entered with blunt dissection. When the epigastric vessels are encountered, they are preserved and retracted. Lateral to the vertebral bodies, the left psoas muscle should be identified. The left common iliac artery and vein should be identified and bluntly swept away from the peritoneum. Additionally, the ureter should be identified and mobilized away from the field. A retractor blade system is then used (**Fig. 2**). A pulse oximeter is attached to the patient's left foot (**Fig. 3**A) and may be monitored during surgery to assess for compromised blood flow during surgery.[24] Adjustment of retractor position may be necessary if a change in the plethysmogram (**Fig. 3**B) is encountered.

The iliac arteries and veins are exposed. The approach to the anterior disk space depends on the ALIF level. At the L2-3 and L3-4 levels, the segmental artery and vein should be divided at each level. The aorta and iliac artery and veins should be mobilized to the right. At the L4-5 level, the L4 segmental artery and vein should be divided and, importantly, the iliolumbar veins should be identified and divided. The latter is at risk for a retraction tear during mobilization of the left common iliac vein, which can result in significant blood loss. The vessels should again be mobilized to the right. The left external iliac artery is at risk of compression from the retractor system during this mobilization. The external iliac pulse should be palpated and the plethysmogram should be closely evaluated with each manipulation of the retractor system. The artery and vein may need to be separated to facilitate mobilization. At the L5-S1 level, the median sacral vessels may be encountered in the midline and should be divided. The retractors provide a working corridor between the iliac arteries and veins. The disk space exposure is preferentially performed with blunt dissection (eg, peanut dissector) to avoid monopolar injury to the hypogastric plexus, minimizing the risk of retrograde ejaculation.

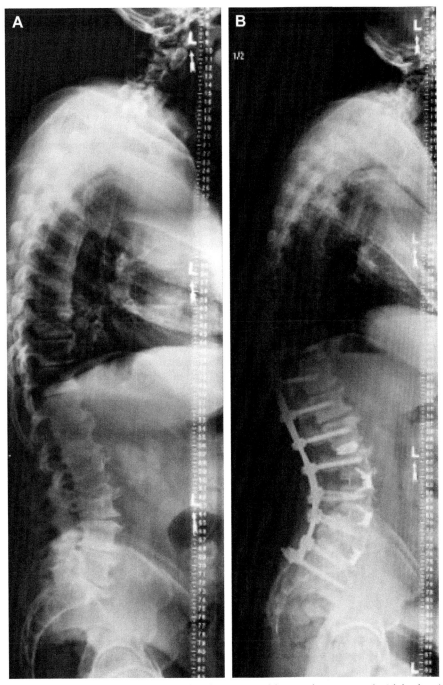

Fig. 1. Preoperative and postoperative radiographs of a 70-year-old man who presented with back pain, scoliosis, and lumbar stenosis. (*A*) Preoperative lateral standing 36-inch plain radiograph demonstrates sagittal imbalance and flat back deformity (SVA 6.2 cm, LL 44°, PI 60°). Deformity correction was accomplished with a multilevel L3–S1 ALIF followed by an open T10-pelvis posterior spinal instrumented fusion. (*B*) Postoperative lateral plain radiograph demonstrates correction of sagittal deformity with restoration of LL appropriate for the respective pelvic incidence (SVA 3.8 cm, LL 60°, PI 60°).

Fluoroscopy should be used to confirm localization. An annulotomy knife is used to enter the disk space with care taken to cut directly along the cephalad and caudally located end plates. Next, a Cobb elevator is placed between the cephalad and caudal space between the disk and end plate and this plane is developed. The disk fragments are then removed with a combination of pituitary

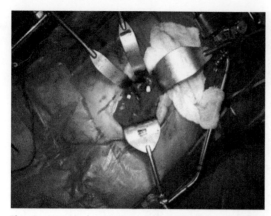

Fig. 2. A typical retractor system used for the ALIF approach.

rongeur and curettes. The end plates are then prepared using a combination of curettes and rasps. If necessary for neural decompression, resection of the posterior longitudinal ligament and any disk fragments may be completed.

Interbody trials are then sequentially inserted into the disk space to serially dilate the disk space height and induce progressive segmental lordosis (**Fig. 4**). Once sufficient disk space height and lordotic correction have been achieved, the appropriate sized implant is chosen. Release of the posterior longitudinal ligament may be necessary to improve foraminal height in patients with foraminal narrowing. The interbody device is then prepared with bone graft (autograft and/or allograft) and/or bone morphogenetic protein to facilitate fusion. In cases where a circumferential procedure is planned with posterior column osteotomies, it is generally recommended that the interbody device be either affixed to the vertebral body using screw fixation to reduce risk of device migration during the posterior approach. It is important to use intraoperative radiography to confirm appropriate graft position and lordotic correction.

After meticulous hemostasis is obtained, the anterior rectus sheath is closed with a running PDS suture. The subdermal and skin layers are closed.

In most cases where substantial restoration of LL is required a circumferential release and fusion is performed either on the same day or as a staged procedure. The posterior instrumented fusion is completed through open or minimally invasive techniques depending on surgeon preference and need for posterior column osteotomy. Some surgeons perform the posterior-release operation (eg, facet release or posterior column osteotomy) as the first stage and perform a subsequent "fill-in" procedure where some additional correction may be achieved.

Complications

Despite the advantages of ALIF, there are recognized risks unique to the anterior approach.[25] These include vascular injury, retrograde ejaculation/sympathectomy effect,[26,27] lymphocele, and ureteral injury. There is also risk of ileus, injury to the viscera, enterocutaneous fistula, retroperitoneal collections, abdominal wall protrusion, and hernia.[28–31] Complications occur in 11% to 24% of patients with 1% to 24% of patients

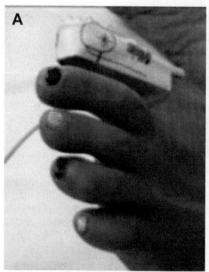

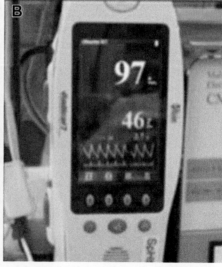

Fig. 3. (*A*) A pulse oximetry device should be placed on the left great toe and the (*B*) plethysmogram monitored closely for changes during manipulation and retraction of the external iliac artery. If changes are encountered, the retraction must be adjusted.

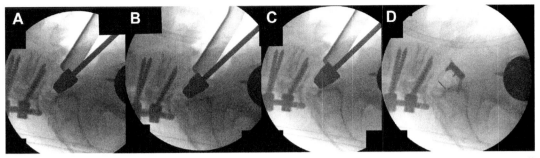

Fig. 4. Intraoperative fluoroscopy during an L5-S1 ALIF. (*A–C*) Sequential insertion of interbody trials to serially dilate the L5-S1 interspace during an L5-S1 ALIF. (*D*) Placement of the final, appropriately sized implant that optimally restores disk space height and segmental lordosis.

experiencing a vascular injury.[22,26,27] Commonly injured vessels include the iliac vein, inferior vena cava, and iliolumbar vein during vessel retraction. Additionally, there is risk of hardware failure and graft subsidence.

PEDICLE SUBTRACTION OSTEOTOMY

Since the initial description by Thomasen[32] in 1985, PSO has been used in the management of fixed sagittal deformity. PSO involves a transpedicular wedge resection extending from the posterior elements and into the anterior cortex of the index vertebral body. PSO permits significant sagittal correction, allowing a correction of 25 to 40° of LL per level,[33,34] a significantly greater increase in per level correction as compared with the Ponte or Smith-Petersen osteotomy and commonly reported, single-level ALIF segmental corrections. Advantages of PSO include the posterior-only approach, avoiding the need for familiarity with the retroperitoneal anatomy or the reliance on an approach surgeon. The primary disadvantage is the technically demanding nature of PSO, involving greater mobilization of neural structures, frequent substantial blood loss, and high rates of rod-fracture, pseudarthrosis, and other complications.[35,36] Despite these disadvantages, in well-selected patients, PSO is associated with significant improvements in pain, self-image, disability, satisfaction, and Scoliosis Research Society outcome scores,[37–39] findings that are durable in long-term follow-up.[40–42] PSO is the procedure of choice for most patients where the anterior spinal column is fused across multiple segments, especially in patients with ankylosing spondylitis or prior surgical interbody fusion.

Indications

PSO is used in patients who have moderate to severe fixed or fused sagittal deformity, who require a minimum of 30° of correction, and in whom multiple

Ponte/Smith-Petersen osteotomies alone would result in inadequate correction. The evidence for PSO for very severe deformity is mixed, with some reports revealing higher rates of postoperative malalignment in those with greater malalignment preoperatively.[43] However, in these patients, PSO, a Schwab grade 3 osteotomy,[44] may be supplemented with multilevel Smith-Peterson osteotomies or may be extended (ie, with additional resection of the cephalad disk [Schwab grade 4 osteotomy]) resulting in closure of the osteotomy wedge onto the adjacent vertebral end plate.

PSO should be used in patients where the characteristics of the deformity benefit from a significant lordotic correction at a single level (contrasted by the multilevel gradual lordosis provided by the multilevel ALIF).

PSO should be considered in patients who have a history of anterior retroperitoneal (abdominal or spinal) surgery because ALIF carries a high risk of complications in these patients. The risk of vascular injury is heightened in redo ALIF cases whereby typical surgical planes are obliterated.[45] Additionally, current or previous osteomyelitis (ie, additional factors leading to inflammation of annular and prevertebral soft tissues) and large osteophyte formation may also increase the risk of vascular injury in an anterior approach.[45] These additional risk factors for vascular injury may lead some to prefer the posterior-only PSO in these cases.

In ASD with concomitant pathology requiring an open posterior approach (eg, significant multilevel spinal stenosis requiring decompression), PSO spares an additional anterior approach. In patients with multiplanar deformity with a component of fixed coronal imbalance, PSO may be done asymmetrically,[46,47] resulting in simultaneous corrections in the sagittal and coronal planes.

Although posterior revision cases are potentially more complex given the need to perform dissection of scar tissue and exposure of previous instrumentation, they should not be considered a general contraindication for PSO. In experienced hands, primary and revision PSO result in similar sagittal deformity correction and complication rates.[48] Prior surgery may restrict deformity correction in some cases. A recent study by Gupta and colleagues[48] of 421 patients undergoing PSO (70 primary patients, 351 revisions patients) found a larger proportion of patients in the primary group were able to achieve optimal PI-LL mismatch compared with the revision group. This may be caused by the greater number of fused segments (particularly the lumbosacral junction) in revision cases, which limited recontouring of the spine.

Technique

Level selection

There are several key considerations for level selection. First, especially in the case of focal sagittal angular deformity, the osteotomy should be performed at the apex of the deformity. Otherwise, we recommend planning a more caudal lumbar level for PSO (eg, L3-S1) for several reasons. The lower level correction more closely approximates physiologic LL[49] and is caudal to the conus medullaris. Additionally, the more caudal level selection results in a larger correction of PT.[50,51] Among the caudal lumbar levels, L3 is commonly chosen for the PSO level because an L4 PSO may stress the L5 nerve root, which could lead to a foot drop.

Osteotomy planning

The goal of the wedge resection is to permit sufficient correction to restore SVA to less than 5 cm while restoring LL to within 10° of PI. An average correction of 30° is generally an appropriate correction goal for PSO; the actual correction can vary among surgeons and is difficult to determine accurately intraoperatively.[38,46]

The approach should be catered to the individual patient to avoid undercorrection or overcorrection. The degree of resection, defined as $\alpha_2-\alpha_1$ (**Fig. 5**),[52] must be diligently planned preoperatively. Multiple planning tools including mathematical methods have been proposed to identify the optimal $\alpha_2-\alpha_1$ preoperatively,[2,34,51,53–55] with varying degrees of accuracy.[52] Aside from the planned focal angular correction, accurate preoperative planning requires an understanding of compensatory changes in the unfused spine and an incorporation of other pelvic alignment parameters, such as PT, and thoracic kyphosis. For example, patients with high PT in conjunction with flat back and sagittal malalignment require larger osteotomies.[56] Failure to anticipate the dynamic changes that occur in the pelvis and cephalad unfused spinal segments after PSO can result in undercorrection of sagittal deformity. Whether geometric, mathematical models are used or not, the general principle is simple: a larger wedge results in a greater correction in LL and, subsequently, sagittal correction.

Surgical technique

The use of two spinal surgeons may be considered and has been shown to decrease operative time and blood loss.[57] Tranexamic acid (TXA) has been used in major spinal surgeries to reduce blood loss and transfusion requirements. The optimal dosing of TXA is controversial because of concerns over the potential for thromboembolic complications. There is increasing evidence that higher doses of TXA are more effective in reducing blood

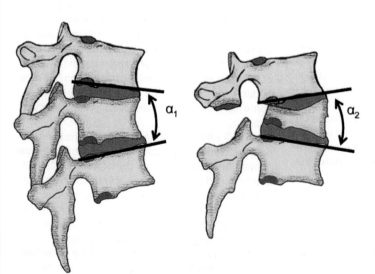

Fig. 5. Measurement of PSO degree of resection, defined as $\alpha_2-\alpha_1$. (*From* Smith JS, Bess S, Shaffrey CI, et al. Dynamic changes of the pelvis and spine are key to predicting postoperative sagittal alignment after pedicle subtraction osteotomy: a critical analysis of preoperative planning techniques. Spine 2012;37(10):845–53; with permission.)

loss.[58] For PSOs, we routinely use a 50 mg/kg loading dose followed by 5 mg/kg/h unless there are strong medical contraindications (eg, history of stroke or recent cardiac stent placement).

Patients are placed prone on a Jackson table and pressure points are padded appropriately. Given the high risk to neural structures, including during the osteotomy correction, the PSO should be performed with motor evoked potential and somatosensory monitoring. Accordingly, anesthetics that blunt motor evoked potential and somatosensory monitoring should be avoided. We prefer a regimen of Propofol, fentanyl, and ketamine and the use of a short-acting paralytic (ie, rocuronium) during endotracheal intubation. A posterior incision is planned allowing adequate visualization of all levels that require instrumentation.

Pedicle screws are then placed cephalad and caudal to the PSO level, skipping the pedicles of the index level. Pedicle screw instrumentation should extend caudally through the pelvis to include iliac fixation. Both upper thoracic (T1-T6) and thoracolumbar levels (T9-L1) have been described for the upper-instrumented vertebra. At least three levels of fixation above the osteotomy is important for cephalad fixation, and three points of fixation distally reduce strain on the instrumentation across the osteotomy. In a study of radiographic outcomes for 165 patients 2 years following lumbar PSO, those with an upper thoracic upper-instrumented vertebra had superior maintenance of sagittal spinopelvic alignment, lower reoperation rates, and lower revision rates for Proximal Junctional Kyphosis but further increases in operative time and blood loss. Screw stimulation or O-arm intraoperative imaging may be performed to ensure accurate screw placement.

Once the posterior bony elements are exposed, a "pedicle-to-pedicle" exposure is required. This results in removal of the spinous processes, the lamina, transverse process, and the superior and inferior facets between the pedicles of the vertebral bodies cephalad and caudal to the PSO vertebral level. The removal of the cephalad and caudal lamina is important because this prevents iatrogenic thecal sac and nerve root impingement on osteotomy closure. The removal of scar in revision cases is likewise important, because the scar can impede smooth buckling of the dura and can potentially cause compression by the scar tissue during osteotomy closure.

Before beginning the osteotomy, a temporary rod or rack is placed to provide stability and avoid premature closure or subluxation of the osteotomy. Next, the pedicles at the index level are resected to the level of the posterior cortex (**Fig. 6**A). After dissection of the psoas away from the lateral vertebral body with a sponge stick or periosteal elevator (**Fig. 6**B), a temporary sponge or spoon-shaped retractor can then be placed medial to the psoas muscle and just ventral to the anterior cortex to provide additional protection and hemostasis.

Then, using a combination of rongeurs and box cutter osteotomes, the vertebral body is decancellated and the lateral vertebral body walls are resected through to the anterior cortex, resulting in a wedge defect in the vertebral body (**Fig. 6**C). The posterior cortex of the vertebral body is then removed with a down-pushing curette to complete the osteotomy. Development of a plane between the ventral thecal sac and the posterior cortex is important before this maneuver to prevent a ventral cerebrospinal fluid leak. Of note, the anterior cortex remains intact, acting as a hinge during the subsequent correction. The cortex additionally affords protection to the anteriorly located great vessels and viscera.

Closure of the osteotomy via extension across the PSO is achieved using several techniques including posterior-based manual compression, manipulation of bolsters, reverse table breaking, rod cantilever technique, and/or additional compression across posterior instrumentation during rod placement (**Fig. 6**D, E). In this stage, avoidance of notch creation in the rod and careful planning and contouring of the rod is important. Precontoured rods may also be used to limit the amount of additional rod bending required. These techniques reduce repeated rod contouring and sharp rod angles and prevent the decrease in resistance of the rod to cyclic loading. Preferential use of cobalt chrome rods may provide the greatest reduction in motion and rod strain at the PSO level,[59] although the evidence is unclear.[60] The use of supplemental satellite or accessory rods has been demonstrated to reduce rod fracture and pseudarthrosis after PSO.[61,62]

It is critical to assess for thecal sac and nerve root impingement during the osteotomy closure via visual inspection and neuromonitoring. The closure can result in subluxation, dural buckling, iatrogenic dorsal impingement, and spinal cord ischemia.[39,63,64] If impingement is noted, a decrease in the magnitude of extension or resection of additional soft tissue or bony structures is performed. To ensure adequate perfusion of the neural elements during osteotomy closure, mean arterial pressures should be maintained greater than 90 mm Hg.

After the instrumentation is locked into final tightness, adequate decortication of the remaining bony surfaces should be completed. Autograft, allograft, bone matrix, and/or bone morphogenetic protein

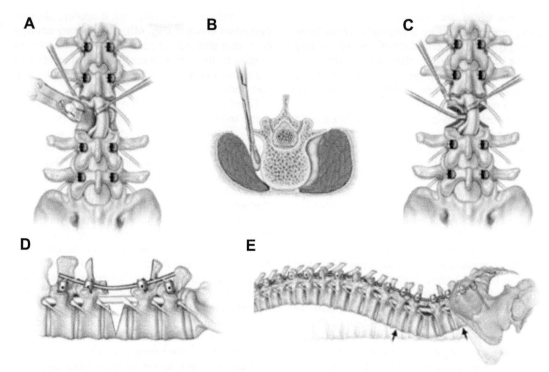

Fig. 6. Illustration of key steps during a pedicle subtraction osteotomy. (*A*) Removal of the posterior elements of the spine should be conducted in a "pedicle-to-pedicle" fashion. The pedicles of the index level are exposed and removed with a rongeur or drill. (*B*) The psoas muscle is dissected away from the lateral aspect of the vertebral body via a sponge stick or a periosteal elevator. (*C*) A wedge resection is created at the level of the pedicle. (*D*) A temporary rod is placed to ensure stability of the spinal column during osteotomy and posterior decompression. (*E*) The osteotomy is closed and lordosis is secured with contoured rods locked into final tightness. (*Adapted from* Mummaneni PV, Dhall SS, Ondra SL, et al. Pedicle subtraction osteotomy. Neurosurgery 2008;63(3 Suppl):171–6; with permission.)

can be used to promote posterolateral fusion. The latter two supplements are especially important in those at increased risk of pseudarthrosis and proximal junctional failure (eg, osteoporosis).

The patient may be placed in a thoracolumbosacral orthosis for 3 to 6 months following the procedure. **Fig. 7** demonstrates preoperative and postoperative lateral radiographs of a patient who underwent PSO for iatrogenic flatback deformity.

PSO may be supplemented with anterior-column support via lumbosacral anterior, transforaminal, and/or lateral interbody fusion.[65] This is performed directly above or below the level of the PSO to provide anterior column support, reduce strain on the rods, and facilitate fusion. Additionally, for fusions that extend to the sacrum, anterior column support should be considered at L5-S1, and the use of iliac fixation.

The configuration of rods during the PSO also has important implications for stability across the PSO level. A four-rod construct[59,61,62,66] is preferred using either accessory or satellite rods. In a study using finite element analysis, there was a 50% primary rod stress reduction (in flexion)

in PSO done with an interbody and four-rod satellite technique compared with a PSO done without an interbody and two-rod construct.[66]

PSO can involve significant blood loss. Thus, techniques to accurately measure volume status, resuscitate the patient, and mitigate blood loss are important, including arterial line and central venous line placement, administration of TXA, use of intraoperative cell saver, and the use of two surgeons may be considered. Judicious transfusion of red blood cells should be used, and preemptive transfusion of cryoprecipitate or fresh frozen plasma should be used in the setting of significant blood loss.

Complications

PSO are associated with high complication rates (as high as 58%[67]).[37,48,64,68] In a study that prospectively collected complication data for 2 years following three-column osteotomy for ASD, 78% of patients had either a minor or major complication.[69] The rate of reoperation was 33%.[69] The most common complications include pseudarthrosis, rod fracture, durotomy, proximal junctional

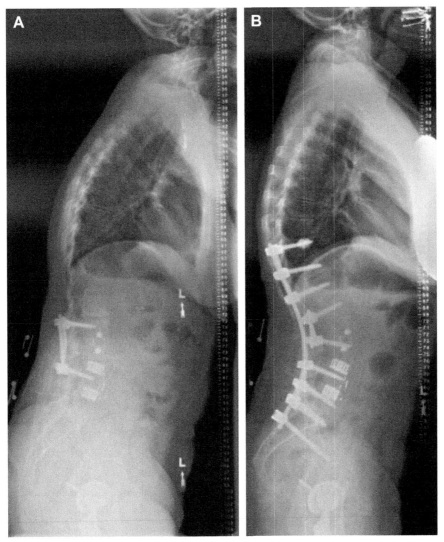

Fig. 7. Preoperative and postoperative radiographs of a 53-year-old woman who presented with severe leg and back pain associated with iatrogenic flat back following a previous L2-4 fusion. (*A*) Preoperative lateral standing 36-inch plain radiograph demonstrates sagittal imbalance and flat back (SVA 15.8 cm, LL 19°, PI 52°). The deformity correction was accomplished with an L2 PSO and T10-pelvis posterior spinal instrumented fusion. (*B*) Postoperative lateral plain radiograph demonstrates correction of the sagittal deformity with restoration of LL appropriate for the respective pelvic incidence (SVA 4.4 cm, LL 57°, PI 52°).

kyphosis, pleural effusion, and deep wound infection.

Neural injury is common, with multiple studies reporting rates around 10%.[37,48,64,67,70] However, in the aforementioned prospective study, the neural injury rate was nearly 30%.

Additionally, suboptimal malalignment is common, with rates reported as high as ~33%.[34] This failure to attain optimal alignment following PSO may result in persistent pain and disability and may require revision surgery.[71]

Other complications include implant prominence; screw breakage; implant loosening; rod dislodgement; screw nerve impingement; adjacent segment disease; and medical complications including postoperative ileus, pulmonary embolism, deep venous thrombosis, urinary tract infection, pneumonia, *Clostridium difficile* infection, sepsis, and even death.

PSO is associated with an increased risk of rod fracture[60] because of the significant stress at the level of the osteotomy. The often high bending angles applied to the rod at the level of the osteotomy produce a shorter fatigue life.[72]

Additional techniques including the use of two deformity surgeons,[57] the use of minimally invasive[73–76] or mini-open techniques,[77] or surgical staging may help to mitigate the risks associated with PSO.

SUMMARY

The use of multilevel ALIF and PSO can achieve a restoration of physiologic LL. Each offers unique advantages and disadvantages. Therefore, the spine surgeon should choose the best technique for a given patient and the type of lordotic correction required.

REFERENCES

1. Mac-Thiong JM, Transfeldt EE, Mehbod AA, et al. Can c7 plumbline and gravity line predict health related quality of life in adult scoliosis? Spine (Phila Pa 1976) 2009;34(15):E519–27.

2. Schwab F, Lafage V, Patel A, et al. Sagittal plane considerations and the pelvis in the adult patient. Spine (Phila Pa 1976) 2009;34(17):1828–33.

3. Schwab F, Patel A, Ungar B, et al. Adult spinal deformity-postoperative standing imbalance: how much can you tolerate? An overview of key parameters in assessing alignment and planning corrective surgery. Spine (Phila Pa 1976) 2010;35(25):2224–31.

4. Booth KC, Bridwell KH, Lenke LG, et al. Complications and predictive factors for the successful treatment of flatback deformity (fixed sagittal imbalance). Spine (Phila Pa 1976) 1999;24(16):1712–20.

5. Casey MP, Asher MA, Jacobs RR, et al. The effect of Harrington rod contouring on lumbar lordosis. Spine (Phila Pa 1976) 1987;12(8):750–3.

6. Farcy JP, Schwab FJ. Management of flatback and related kyphotic decompensation syndromes. Spine (Phila Pa 1976) 1997;22(20):2452–7.

7. Rothenfluh DA, Mueller DA, Rothenfluh E, et al. Pelvic incidence-lumbar lordosis mismatch predisposes to adjacent segment disease after lumbar spinal fusion. Eur Spine J 2015;24(6):1251–8.

8. Umehara S, Zindrick MR, Patwardhan AG, et al. The biomechanical effect of postoperative hypolordosis in instrumented lumbar fusion on instrumented and adjacent spinal segments. Spine (Phila Pa 1976) 2000;25(13):1617–24.

9. Ames CP, Smith JS, Scheer JK, et al. Impact of spinopelvic alignment on decision making in deformity surgery in adults: a review. J Neurosurg Spine 2012;16(6):547–64.

10. Bradford DS, Tay BK, Hu SS. Adult scoliosis: surgical indications, operative management, complications, and outcomes. Spine (Phila Pa 1976) 1999;24(24):2617–29.

11. Glassman SD, Berven S, Bridwell K, et al. Correlation of radiographic parameters and clinical symptoms in adult scoliosis. Spine (Phila Pa 1976) 2005;30(6):682–8.

12. Glassman SD, Bridwell K, Dimar JR, et al. The impact of positive sagittal balance in adult spinal deformity. Spine (Phila Pa 1976) 2005;30(18):2024–9.

13. Schwab FJ, Blondel B, Bess S, et al. Radiographical spinopelvic parameters and disability in the setting of adult spinal deformity: a prospective multicenter analysis. Spine (Phila Pa 1976) 2013;38(13):E803–12.

14. Le Huec JC, Cogniet A, Demezon H, et al. Insufficient restoration of lumbar lordosis and FBI index following pedicle subtraction osteotomy is an indicator of likely mechanical complication. Eur Spine J 2015;24(Suppl 1):S112–20.

15. Hsieh PC, Koski TR, O'Shaughnessy BA, et al. Anterior lumbar interbody fusion in comparison with transforaminal lumbar interbody fusion: implications for the restoration of foraminal height, local disc angle, lumbar lordosis, and sagittal balance. J Neurosurg Spine 2007;7(4):379–86.

16. Dahl BT, Harris JA, Gudipally M, et al. Kinematic efficacy of supplemental anterior lumbar interbody fusion at lumbosacral levels in thoracolumbosacral deformity correction with and without pedicle subtraction osteotomy at L3: an in vitro cadaveric study. Eur Spine J 2017;26(11):2773–81.

17. Bae J, Theologis AA, Strom R, et al. Comparative analysis of 3 surgical strategies for adult spinal deformity with mild to moderate sagittal imbalance. J Neurosurg Spine 2017;28(1):1–10.

18. Suh LR, Jo DJ, Kim SM, et al. A surgical option for multilevel anterior lumbar interbody fusion with ponte osteotomy to achieve optimal lumbar lordosis and sagittal balance. J Korean Neurosurg Soc 2012;52(4):365–71.

19. Kadam A, Wigner N, Saville P, et al. Overpowering posterior lumbar instrumentation and fusion with hyperlordotic anterior lumbar interbody cages followed by posterior revision: a preliminary feasibility study. J Neurosurg Spine 2017;27(6):1–11.

20. Wigner N, Kadam A, Saville P, et al. Can posterior lumbar instrumentation and fusion be overpowered by anterior lumbar fusion with hyperlordotic cages? A cadaveric study. Glob Spine J 2017;7(7):689–95.

21. Asha MJ, Choksey MS, Shad A, et al. The role of the vascular surgeon in anterior lumbar spine surgery. Br J Neurosurg 2012;26(4):499–503.

22. Mobbs RJ, Phan K, Daly D, et al. Approach-related complications of anterior lumbar interbody fusion: results of a combined spine and vascular surgical team. Glob Spine J 2016;6(2):147–54.

23. Tropiano P, Giorgi H, Faure A, et al. Surgical techniques for lumbo-sacral fusion. Orthop Traumatol Surg Res 2017;103(1S):S151–9.

24. Brau SA, Delamarter RB, Schiffman ML, et al. Vascular injury during anterior lumbar surgery. Spine J 2004;4(4):409–12.

25. Faciszewski T, Winter RB, Lonstein JE, et al. The surgical and medical perioperative complications of anterior spinal fusion surgery in the thoracic and lumbar spine in adults. A review of 1223 procedures. Spine (Phila Pa 1976) 1995;20(14):1592–9.

26. Garg J, Woo K, Hirsch J, et al. Vascular complications of exposure for anterior lumbar interbody fusion. J Vasc Surg 2010;51(4):946 50 [discussion: 950].

27. McDonnell MF, Glassman SD, Dimar JR 2nd, et al. Perioperative complications of anterior procedures on the spine. J Bone Joint Surg Am 1996;78(6):839–47.

28. Giang G, Mobbs R, Phan S, et al. Evaluating outcomes of stand-alone anterior lumbar interbody fusion: a systematic review. World Neurosurg 2017;104:259–71.

29. Mobbs RJ, Phan K, Malham G, et al. Lumbar interbody fusion: techniques, indications and comparison of interbody fusion options including PLIF, TLIF, MI-TLIF, OLIF/ATP, LLIF and ALIF. J Spine Surg 2015;1(1):2–18.

30. Phan K, Thayaparan GK, Mobbs RJ. Anterior lumbar interbody fusion versus transforaminal lumbar interbody fusion: systematic review and meta-analysis. Br J Neurosurg 2015;29(5):705–11.

31. Teng I, Han J, Phan K, et al. A meta-analysis comparing ALIF, PLIF, TLIF and LLIF. J Clin Neurosci 2017;44:11–7.

32. Thomasen E. Vertebral osteotomy for correction of kyphosis in ankylosing spondylitis. Clin Orthop Relat Res 1985;(194):142–52.

33. Bridwell KH, Lewis SJ, Lenke LG, et al. Pedicle subtraction osteotomy for the treatment of fixed sagittal imbalance. J Bone Joint Surg Am 2003;85-A(3):454–63.

34. Rose PS, Bridwell KH, Lenke LG, et al. Role of pelvic incidence, thoracic kyphosis, and patient factors on sagittal plane correction following pedicle subtraction osteotomy. Spine (Phila Pa 1976) 2009;34(8):785–91.

35. Bridwell KH, Lewis SJ, Rinella A, et al. Pedicle subtraction osteotomy for the treatment of fixed sagittal imbalance. Surgical technique. J Bone Joint Surg Am 2004;86-A(Suppl 1):44–50.

36. Wang MY, Berven SH. Lumbar pedicle subtraction osteotomy. Neurosurgery 2007;60(2 Suppl 1):ONS140–6 [discussion: ONS146].

37. Bridwell KH, Lewis SJ, Edwards C, et al. Complications and outcomes of pedicle subtraction osteotomies for fixed sagittal imbalance. Spine (Phila Pa 1976) 2003;28(18):2093–101.

38. Barrey C, Perrin G, Michel F, et al. Pedicle subtraction osteotomy in the lumbar spine: indications, technical aspects, results and complications. Eur J Orthop Surg Traumatol 2014;24(Suppl 1):S21–30.

39. Yang BP, Ondra SL, Chen LA, et al. Clinical and radiographic outcomes of thoracic and lumbar pedicle subtraction osteotomy for fixed sagittal imbalance. J Neurosurg Spine 2006;5(1):9–17.

40. Kim KT, Lee SH, Suk KS, et al. Outcome of pedicle subtraction osteotomies for fixed sagittal imbalance of multiple etiologies: a retrospective review of 140 patients. Spine (Phila Pa 1976) 2012;37(19):1667–75.

41. Kim YJ, Bridwell KH, Lenke LG, et al. Results of lumbar pedicle subtraction osteotomies for fixed sagittal imbalance: a minimum 5-year follow-up study. Spine (Phila Pa 1976) 2007;32(20):2189–97.

42. O'Neill KR, Lenke LG, Bridwell KH, et al. Clinical and radiographic outcomes after 3-column osteotomies with 5-year follow-up. Spine (Phila Pa 1976) 2014;39(5):424–32.

43. Schwab FJ, Patel A, Shaffrey CI, et al. Sagittal realignment failures following pedicle subtraction osteotomy surgery: are we doing enough? Clinical article. J Neurosurg Spine 2012;16(6):539–46.

44. Schwab F, Blondel B, Chay E, et al. The comprehensive anatomical spinal osteotomy classification. Neurosurgery 2014;74(1):112–20 [discussion: 120].

45. Fantini GA, Pappou IP, Girardi FP, et al. Major vascular injury during anterior lumbar spinal surgery: incidence, risk factors, and management. Spine (Phila Pa 1976) 2007;32(24):2751–8.

46. Bridwell KH. Decision making regarding Smith-Petersen vs. pedicle subtraction osteotomy vs. vertebral column resection for spinal deformity. Spine (Phila Pa 1976) 2006;31(19 Suppl):S171–8.

47. Chan AK, Lau D, Osorio JA, et al. Asymmetric pedicle subtraction osteotomy for adult spinal deformity with coronal plane imbalance: complications, radiographic, and surgical outcomes. 33nd Annual Meeting of the Section on Disorders of the Spine and Peripheral Nerves. Las Vegas, NV, Mar 8-11, 2017.

48. Gupta MC, Ferrero E, Mundis G, et al. Pedicle subtraction osteotomy in the revision versus primary adult spinal deformity patient: is there a difference in correction and complications? Spine (Phila Pa 1976) 2015;40(22):E1169–75.

49. Bernhardt M, Bridwell KH. Segmental analysis of the sagittal plane alignment of the normal thoracic and lumbar spines and thoracolumbar junction. Spine (Phila Pa 1976) 1989;14(7):717–21.

50. Berjano P, Aebi M. Pedicle subtraction osteotomies (PSO) in the lumbar spine for sagittal deformities. Eur Spine J 2015;24(Suppl 1):S49–57.

51. Lafage V, Schwab F, Vira S, et al. Spino-pelvic parameters after surgery can be predicted: a preliminary formula and validation of standing alignment. Spine (Phila Pa 1976) 2011;36(13):1037–45.

52. Smith JS, Bess S, Shaffrey CI, et al. Dynamic changes of the pelvis and spine are key to predicting postoperative sagittal alignment after pedicle subtraction osteotomy: a critical analysis of

preoperative planning techniques. Spine (Phila Pa 1976) 2012;37(10):845–53.

53. Kim YJ, Bridwell KH, Lenke LG, et al. An analysis of sagittal spinal alignment following long adult lumbar instrumentation and fusion to L5 or S1: can we predict ideal lumbar lordosis? Spine (Phila Pa 1976) 2006;31(20):2343–52.

54. Lafage V, Bharucha NJ, Schwab F, et al. Multicenter validation of a formula predicting postoperative spinopelvic alignment. J Neurosurg Spine 2012;16(1): 15–21.

55. Ondra SL, Marzouk S, Koski T, et al. Mathematical calculation of pedicle subtraction osteotomy size to allow precision correction of fixed sagittal deformity. Spine (Phila Pa 1976) 2006;31(25):E973–9.

56. Lafage V, Blondel B, Smith JS, et al. Preoperative planning for pedicle subtraction osteotomy: does pelvic tilt matter? Spine Deform 2014;2(5):358–66.

57. Ames CP, Barry JJ, Keshavarzi S, et al. Perioperative outcomes and complications of pedicle subtraction osteotomy in cases with single versus two attending surgeons. Spine Deform 2013;1(1):51–8.

58. Xie J, Lenke LG, Li T, et al. Preliminary investigation of high-dose tranexamic acid for controlling intraoperative blood loss in patients undergoing spine correction surgery. Spine J 2015;15(4):647–54.

59. Hallager DW, Gehrchen M, Dahl B, et al. Use of supplemental short pre-contoured accessory rods and cobalt chrome alloy posterior rods reduces primary rod strain and range of motion across the pedicle subtraction osteotomy level: an in vitro biomechanical study. Spine (Phila Pa 1976) 2016;41(7):E388–95.

60. Smith JS, Shaffrey E, Klineberg E, et al. Prospective multicenter assessment of risk factors for rod fracture following surgery for adult spinal deformity. J Neurosurg Spine 2014;21(6):994–1003.

61. Gupta S, Eksi MS, Ames CP, et al. A novel 4-Rod technique offers potential to reduce rod breakage and pseudarthrosis in pedicle subtraction osteotomies for adult spinal deformity correction. Oper Neurosurg (Hagerstown) 2018;14(4):449–56.

62. Hyun SJ, Lenke LG, Kim YC, et al. Comparison of standard 2-rod constructs to multiple-rod constructs for fixation across 3-column spinal osteotomies. Spine (Phila Pa 1976) 2014;39(22):1899–904.

63. Ahn UM, Ahn NU, Buchowski JM, et al. Functional outcome and radiographic correction after spinal osteotomy. Spine (Phila Pa 1976) 2002;27(12): 1303–11.

64. Buchowski JM, Bridwell KH, Lenke LG, et al. Neurologic complications of lumbar pedicle subtraction osteotomy: a 10-year assessment. Spine (Phila Pa 1976) 2007;32(20):2245–52.

65. Deviren V, Tang JA, Scheer JK, et al. Construct rigidity after fatigue loading in pedicle subtraction

osteotomy with or without adjacent interbody structural cages. Glob Spine J 2012;2(4):213–20.

66. Januszewski J, Beckman JM, Harris JE, et al. Biomechanical study of rod stress after pedicle subtraction osteotomy versus anterior column reconstruction: a finite element study. Surg Neurol Int 2017;8:207.

67. Cho KJ, Bridwell KH, Lenke LG, et al. Comparison of Smith-Petersen versus pedicle subtraction osteotomy for the correction of fixed sagittal imbalance. Spine (Phila Pa 1976) 2005;30(18):2030–7 [discussion: 2038].

68. Schwab FJ, Hawkinson N, Lafage V, et al. Risk factors for major peri-operative complications in adult spinal deformity surgery: a multi-center review of 953 consecutive patients. Eur Spine J 2012;21(12): 2603–10.

69. Smith JS, Shaffrey CI, Klineberg E, et al. Complication rates associated with 3-column osteotomy in 82 adult spinal deformity patients: retrospective review of a prospectively collected multicenter consecutive series with 2-year follow-up. J Neurosurg Spine 2017;27(4):444–57.

70. Kelly MP, Lenke LG, Shaffrey CI, et al. Evaluation of complications and neurological deficits with three-column spine reconstructions for complex spinal deformity: a retrospective Scoli-RISK-1 study. Neurosurg Focus 2014;36(5):E17.

71. Gottfried ON, Daubs MD, Patel AA, et al. Spinopelvic parameters in postfusion flatback deformity patients. Spine J 2009;9(8):639–47.

72. Tang JA, Leasure JM, Smith JS, et al. Effect of severity of rod contour on posterior rod failure in the setting of lumbar pedicle subtraction osteotomy (PSO): a biomechanical study. Neurosurgery 2013; 72(2):276–82 [discussion: 283].

73. Dangelmajer S, Zadnik PL, Rodriguez ST, et al. Minimally invasive spine surgery for adult degenerative lumbar scoliosis. Neurosurg Focus 2014;36(5):E7.

74. Kanter AS, Tempel ZJ, Ozpinar A, et al. A review of minimally invasive procedures for the treatment of adult spinal deformity. Spine (Phila Pa 1976) 2016; 41(Suppl 8):S59–65.

75. Mummaneni PV, Shaffrey CI, Lenke LG, et al. The minimally invasive spinal deformity surgery algorithm: a reproducible rational framework for decision making in minimally invasive spinal deformity surgery. Neurosurg Focus 2014;36(5):E6.

76. Mummaneni PV, Tu TH, Ziewacz JE, et al. The role of minimally invasive techniques in the treatment of adult spinal deformity. Neurosurg Clin N Am 2013; 24(2):231–48.

77. Wang MY, Bordon G. Mini-open pedicle subtraction osteotomy as a treatment for severe adult spinal deformities: case series with initial clinical and radiographic outcomes. J Neurosurg Spine 2016;24(5):769–76.

The Nuances of Pedicle Subtraction Osteotomies

Sachin Gupta, BS[a], Munish C. Gupta, MD[b],*

KEYWORDS

- Pedicle subtraction osteotomy • Four-rod technique • Deformity • Rod failures • Pseudoarthrosis

KEY POINTS

- Pedicle subtraction osteotomy (PSO) can be used in a rigid, previously fused spine.
- Consider using the 4-rod technique to decrease rod failures.
- Be aware of neurologic complications and use neuromonitoring.

INTRODUCTION

The pedicle subtraction osteotomy (PSO), first described by Thomasen,[1] is an extremely useful technique for the treatment of adult spinal deformity.[1] In the setting of severely rigid spinal deformities and in the previously fused spine, the PSO can provide correction in the sagittal plane of up to 30° to 40° without the need for a combined anterior and posterior approach.[2] In addition, this posterior-only osteotomy can provide significant correction without lengthening the anterior column, unlike its close relative the Smith-Peterson osteotomy.[2–5]

Thomasen's[1] first description of the PSO involved a series of 11 patients with ankylosing spondylitis for which he used a wedge posterior osteotomy of the second lumbar vertebra to restore lordosis. The procedure itself involves a 3-column osteotomy with the transpedicular wedge resection extending from the posterior elements through the vertebral body. However, the anterior cortex is left intact, allowing for the closure of the wedge and shortening of the posterior column without lengthening the anterior column. Keeping the anterior cortex intact avoids injury to the anterior abdominal viscera and major vessels including the aorta.

Nevertheless, its success in providing such great sagittal correction and restoration of lumbar lordosis comes with a price. The PSO is traditionally performed with 2 rods, which experience a significant amount of stress across the apex of the osteotomy at the wedge closure where the correction is achieved. Smith[6] and his group reported rod failure rates of up to 15.8% in 114 patients treated with PSO. In a previous study, the senior author has developed and compared a novel 4-rod technique to the traditional 2-rod technique in an effort to avoid such failures.[7] With further description later, the technique allows for distribution of the stress along 2 smaller rods placed immediately above and below the osteotomy sites with 2 additional long rods that bridge across the osteotomy without being connected to the smaller rods. In this manner, this configuration decreases the vulnerability of the rods for rod fracture and reduces the rate of pseudoarthrosis.

Technique

Indications for the PSO include fixed sagittal malalignment and prior anterior column fusion (**Table 1**).[8] Decision-making regarding the PSO level depends on several factors. It is more commonly performed below the conus in the lumbar spine to reduce neurologic complications from thecal sac manipulation and wedge closure. However, it can be performed at the thoracic or cervical

Disclosure: Dr M. Gupta owns personal J&J and P&G stock. An OMeGA grant and AO Spine North American grants paid to institution. S. Gupta has nothing to disclose.
a Department of Orthopaedic Surgery, The George Washington University, 2300 Street NW, Washington, DC 20052, USA; b Washington University School of Medicine, Campus Box 8233, 660 Euclid Avenue, St Louis, MO 63110, USA
* Corresponding author.
E-mail address: munishgupta@wustl.edu

Neurosurg Clin N Am 29 (2018) 355–363
https://doi.org/10.1016/j.nec.2018.03.001
1042-3680/18/© 2018 Elsevier Inc. All rights reserved.

Table 1
Indications and contraindications for pedicle subtraction osteotomies

Indications	Contraindications
>25° correction of lordosis desired	Medical contraindications
Spine stiffness (unable to achieve correction in extension radiographs)	Poor bone quality, which may result in failure to close or fuse across osteotomy site
Circumferential fusion over multiple segments	Normal sagittal or coronal alignment
Coronal malalignment in a fused spine	Mobile anterior column that can be treated with combined anteroposterior approach or posterior-based Ponte osteotomies
>10 cm sagittal imbalance	More than 40° of correction (may require extended Pedicle subtraction osteotomy (PSO) or vertebral column resection)

level in certain cases, such as posttraumatic kyphosis. In these cases, retraction of the thecal sac should be avoided.

The level of the PSO itself should depend on the location and the type of the spinal deformity. If patients have a focal fixed-angled sagittal deformity, the PSO should be performed at the level of the kyphosis. However, in the absence of such kyphosis, a lumbar PSO should be performed.

Careful planning beginning outside the operating room is paramount to achieving improved efficiency of the procedure itself, improved operative time, decreased blood loss, and less complications.

EXPOSURE

The surgeon should take great care in providing extensive, meticulous exposure with excellent hemostasis. During exposure, one should preserve the interspinous and supraspinous ligaments in the area of the upper instrumented vertebra. This preservation is performed to prevent proximal junctional kyphosis (PJK), as described by Anderson and his colleagues.[9] With careful attention to the anatomic variation in size, angulation, and rotation of the pedicles, screws are then placed above

and below the planned level of the PSO at multiple levels, with 2 being the minimum.

DECOMPRESSION

The posterior laminectomies and decompression are then performed. At the level of the PSO, a complete laminectomy extending through the bilateral pars interarticularis is performed in addition to bilateral facetectomies. However, superior and inferior to the level of the PSO, a partial laminectomy is performed through the bilateral pars interarticularis. Centrally, decompression is achieved with resection of the ligamentum flavum. In the case of revision laminectomies, one should take care removing the scar tissue above the thecal sac. Removing the scar allows the dura to have multiple buckles rather than one stiff area producing a single buckle, which can cause cauda equina compression. At the level of the PSO, the bone surrounding the pedicle is completely removed, including the transverse process. This removal should provide exposure of the 4 nerve roots bilaterally (**Fig. 1**). At the level of the pedicle, the cobb elevator is used to expose the vertebral body on both sides. If the segmental vessels are encountered, bipolar cautery is used to control the bleeding. The plane between the lateral aspect of the vertebral body and the adjacent soft tissue is then developed and maintained with the use of sponges or retractors. This action allows for adequate visualization of the bony anatomy, including the vertebral body. At this point, the posterior retractors are placed. Using nerve root retractors to protect each individual nerve root, the pedicle is decancellated and the vertebral body is hollowed out using a curette. The wall of the pedicle is then resected using a rongeur.

WEDGE OSTEOTOMY

Using an osteotome, a preplanned wedge is made with wider resection posteriorly, allowing for

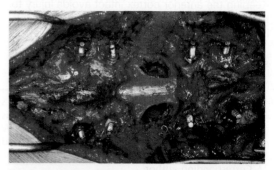

Fig. 1. Exposure of the 4 nerve roots and 6 pedicles is essential before performing the pedicle subtraction osteotomy.

creation of the proper wedge. If necessary, fluoroscopic guidance can be used to maintain orientation when creating such a wedge. If a wedge is not created, this will not improve the lordosis or sagittal alignment but instead will result in shortening of the entire column. One must also take care to resect laterally from the walls of the vertebral body to prevent impingement on closure. The spoon retractors should be placed with care to separate the psoas from the vertebra body side walls and not left in place for a long time.

In this manner, the anterior cortex remains preserved, which allows for decreased risk of injury to the anterior vessels and viscera. During the osteotomy, one must take care to continuously protect the nerve roots and thecal sac with the appropriate nerve root retractors in addition to providing hemostasis control with the use of hemostatic agents and sponges. When performing an osteotomy on one side, a rod should be placed above and below the osteotomy site; the process should be repeated on the other side. When decancellating the vertebral body, one must take care to begin with creating a thin posterior cortical wall. Then a Woodson or a curved freer can be used to remove any dural adhesions to the posterior wall to prevent injury to the anterior portion of the dura. Once the resection of the lateral walls is complete, a Woodson or a posterior body wall impactor can be used to fracture the posterior wall into the cavity created and these elements can be resected using a Leksell or pituitary rongeur. In addition, asymmetric PSOs can be performed in the cases of kyphoscoliotic deformities, allowing for correction in the coronal plane on wedge closure.

OSTEOTOMY CLOSURE

Before obtaining closure of the osteotomy, care must be taken to remove any remaining bony fragments than might compress the exiting nerves because the 2 adjacent exiting nerves will now share a newly created super foramen on each side. A table that may bend the torso in extension can be very useful in closing the osteotomy. Closing the osteotomy with the help of the table can be more useful than closing the osteotomy by compression across the screws above and below the osteotomy. During closure, with the help of neuromonitoring, the neural elements are carefully accounted for. If no neuromonitoring changes are recorded and the nerve roots are free of any impingement from bone or soft tissue, the surgeon can then place the final rods and perform final tightening.

In this manner, the wedge osteotomy can be successfully closed and the correction is

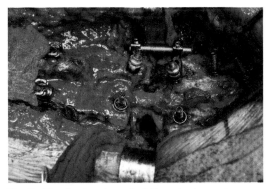

Fig. 2. The short rods control the osteotomy closure as well as prevent translation while finishing the osteotomy.

maintained by the short rods connecting the immediate adjacent levels (**Fig. 2**). The long rods are then placed along the length of the instrumented fusion and are not connected to the screws attached to the short rods (**Fig. 3**). This placement avoids the need for severe angular bending of the long rods, which can weaken the rods, make them vulnerable to rod fractures, and predispose patients to pseudoarthrosis. If there is any concerning change in the neurophysiologic monitoring, the closure should be stopped and reversed to protect the neural elements and further decompression and resection of the bony elements may be necessary.

FINISHING STEPS

The procedure is then completed with decortication with a high-speed drill followed by placement of harvested bone graft or the off-label use of recombinant human bone morphogenetic protein 2. Drains are then placed, and closure of the wound is then performed. A case example is presented in **Figs. 4–7**.

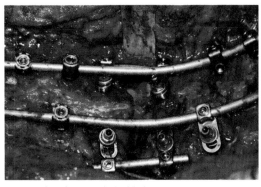

Fig. 3. The short rods hold the osteotomy correction during placement of the long rods and are independent of the long rods.

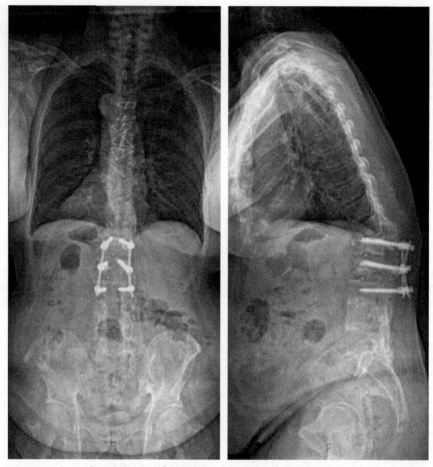

Fig. 4. These preoperative radiographs are of a 65-year-old man with 4 prior spine surgeries in 1998, 2008, 2015, and 2016. He had a fusion at L4-L5 and developed footdrop on the right side. The fusion was extended to L3 and then extended again to L1. The fusion was revised from L1 to L3 because of screw cut out. He presented in the clinic with junctional failure above L1.

COMPLICATIONS

Although the PSO can provide excellent correction in the treatment of rigid curves and in previously fused spines, it is not without its complications. The major complications well known to adult spinal deformity surgeons who perform this procedure include high intraoperative blood loss, neurologic deficits, and pseudoarthrosis.

BLOOD LOSS

Minimizing blood loss is essential with decreasing postoperative complications following pedicle subtraction osteotomies. Although paying close attention to adequate hemostasis during the procedure is beneficial, others have found a solution to decrease blood loss with minimally invasive techniques. Wang and his colleagues[10] demonstrated decreased blood loss with improved

deformity parameters. Despite these encouraging results, further studies with greater follow-up are necessary to further determine the efficacy of these newly developed techniques.[10–12] The use of tranexamic acid has decreased the blood loss in these osteotomy procedures.[13]

NEUROLOGIC DEFICITS

Surgeons who perform pedicle subtraction osteotomies are no stranger to neurologic complications ranging from mild radiculopathies to cauda equina and cord injury. Most importantly, one must use visualization of the nerve roots and adequate intraoperative neuromonitoring during closure of the wedge osteotomy to prevent neurologic injury. Buchowski and colleagues[14] reported a neurologic deficit of 11.1%, with 2.8% permanent deficits. In addition, performing PSOs in the cervical spine, such as at the level of C7 or T1, can result

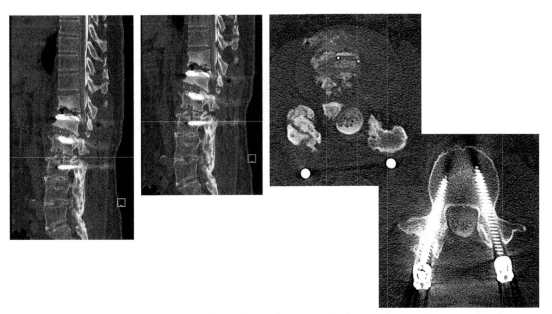

Fig. 5. The computed tomography scan shows bone fragments in the canal as well as pseudoarthroses at multiple levels.

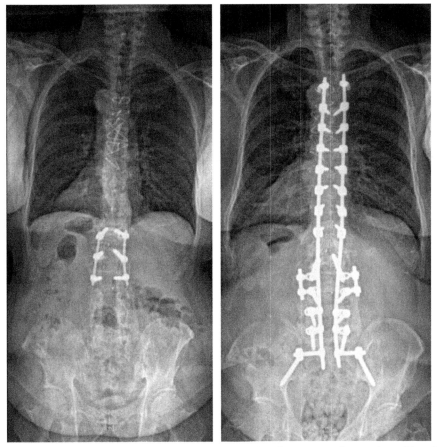

Fig. 6. Preoperative and postoperative PA radiographs demonstrating the amount of correction achieved with the 4-rod technique. PSO allows for correction of the flat back as well as extension of the fusion into the thoracic spine.

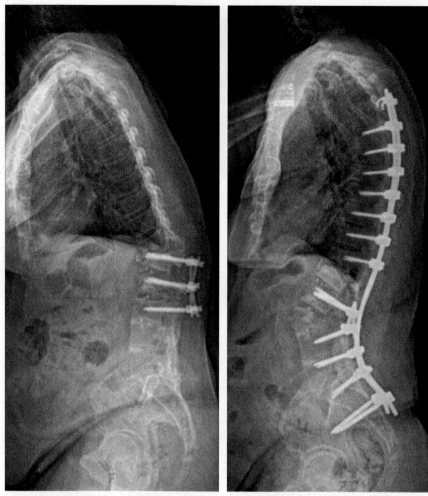

Fig. 7. Preoperative and postoperative *lateral* radiographs demonstrating the amount of correction achieved with the 4-rod technique. PSO allows for correction of the flat back as well as extension of the fusion into the thoracic spine.

in C8 radiculopathies.[15,16] It is critical to use multimodal neuromonitoring during the procedure and have a standardized protocol to respond to abnormal neuromonitoring signals.

PSEUDOARTHROSIS

Pseudoarthrosis is a complication that can present early or delayed. Risk factors include thoracolumbar kyphosis, thoracoabdominal approach, positive sagittal balance of 5 cm or greater at 8 weeks postoperatively, older age (>55 years) at surgery, incomplete sacropelvic fixation, lumbar lordosis change greater than 30°, postoperative thoracic kyphosis greater than 50°, postoperative sacral slope of 30° or less, prior pseudoarthrosis, prior lumbar decompression, prior radiation to the lumbar spine, inflammatory/neurologic disorders.[17–19]

In 2014, Smith and colleagues[17] suggested using alternative instrumentation techniques to prevent rod fractures and pseudoarthroses. Hyun and colleagues[20] demonstrated that using multiple rods compared with 2 rods across the PSO decreased rod fractures. Hallager and colleagues[21] found reduction in strain with the placement of accessory cobalt-chrome rods across the PSO site in addition to interbody spacers adjacent to the PSO site. Others, including Luca and colleagues,[22] have tried different types of rods, finding that larger titanium rods had less stress across PSO sites compared with smaller titanium and cobalt chrome rods. Nevertheless, Tang and colleagues[23] were able to demonstrate that contouring the rods significantly decreases the fatigue life; it was this significant rod contouring across the PSO site that was leading to the rod breakages. This finding led Gupta and colleagues[7] to demonstrate using a 4-rod technique where the 2 long rods bridged over the osteotomy did not have to be contoured as much as previously, resulting in less rod fractures. The satellite rods were able to maintain the correction at the level of the osteotomy. This technique was different from the multi-rod constructs used in the past by Hyun and colleagues[20] because the rods were not connected and the amount of stress on the construct was reduced because of less contouring, which is what decreased the rate of rod fractures and pseudoarthrosis.

NUANCES FOR THE PEDICLE SUBTRACTION OSTEOTOMY
Decompression

It is paramount for surgeons to perform a wide decompression for the visualization of the 4 nerve roots and 6 pedicles before beginning the osteotomy. The entire fusion mass laterally has to be removed as part of the decompression. In addition, any tissue or bone around the pedicles has to be removed and the nerve roots must be traced all the way around the pedicles into the soft tissue.

Closure Technique

Various methods of closing the PSO have been described. There is a cantilever technique that anchors the rods proximally and then with force approximates the rods into the distal screws. The cantilever technique closes the osteotomy, as the rods are seated into the distal screws. The danger of the cantilever technique is the loss of fixation that can happen on the proximal anchors. The other disadvantage is the loss of contour of the rod during correction. This loss decreases the amount of correction that can be achieved. In addition, the sharp contour of the rod across the apex of the osteotomy makes it vulnerable at the PSO site.

The second method commonly used is the compression of the osteotomy site using the screws around the osteotomy site. This technique heavily depends on the quality of the fixation above and below the osteotomy site. The PSO is commonly performed in a previously fused spine. The fused segments with instrumentation have stress shielding and frequently develop osteopenia. This point should be kept in mind when placing compression across the screws that could easily break the pedicle or plow through the vertebral body.

The third technique uses the table that bends the torso in extension. This technique is preferred by the senior author because it can help gain correction without jeopardizing the fixation of the pedicle screws. The closure of the bed can be gradual allowing for checking the neural elements periodically and judging the appropriate amount of correction. Asymmetric closure of the wedge is also possible with this technique. The temporary rods are not only used to guide the correction and prevent catastrophic translation, but also can allow the contralateral side to gain a large compression and greater correction. The short rods are used to control the closure are then tightened. The long rods are then placed only after the desired correction has been acquired. The long rods bridge across the osteotomy site and are not connected to the short rods. Therefore, they are not vulnerable to rod failure. The advantage of the satellite rods is to give better control and greater correction at the osteotomy site while preventing long-term pseudoarthrosis and instrumentation failure at the osteotomy site. A classification of the multiple rods that can be used across the osteotomy site has been developed to address the confusion around the use of the multiple rods (**Fig. 8**).

Adequate Correction

Correction at the osteotomy site can be maximized by using the grade 3 and 4 PSO as needed. The difference between grade 3 and grade 4 involves the additional removal of the disk space proximally. The removal of the disk space allows for greater shortening of the middle and posterior columns but maintains the length of the anterior column. The use of the angulated table also uses the osteotomy as a fulcrum to achieve greater sagittal vertical axis (SVA) correction rather than the triangular wedge approximation of the vertebral body. The center of the correction is the foramen as the torso is brought back posteriorly to correct the SVA.

The correction needed in terms of SVA and lumbar lordosis can be judged by pelvic incidence and the thoracic kyphosis. In general, the apex of the lumbar lordosis can be placed at the L3 or L4 vertebral body. The L4 PSO may give greater SVA correction but has the disadvantage of not having as many distal fixation points as shown by Lafage and colleagues.[24] The other advantage is that it provides lordosis closer to L4-S1 where approximately two-thirds of the lordosis is usually present. On the other hand, if the PSO is performed at L3 with an anterior lumbar interbody fusion at L5-S1, greater lordosis and harmonious correction can be achieved. Excess lordosis, however, should be avoided because it can increase the incidence of PJK. Recently, others have demonstrated that age-appropriate correction of lordosis can be performed to decrease PJK and have developed the Global Alignment and Proportion score that uses pelvic version (the measured minus the ideal sacral slope), relative lumbar lordosis (the measured minus the ideal lumbar lordosis), lordosis distribution

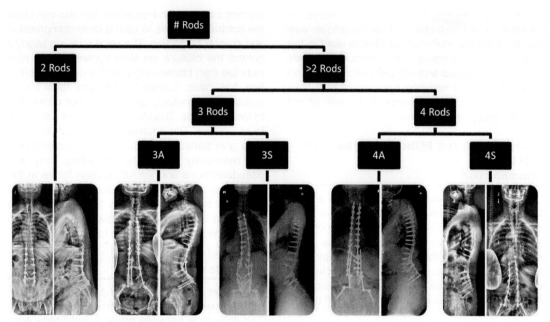

Fig. 8. Classification describing the use of multiple rod constructs. A, accessory; S, satellite.

index (the L4-S1 lordosis divided by the L1-S1 lordosis multiplied by 100), relative spinopelvic alignment (the measured minus the ideal global tilt), and an age as a way to prevent mechanical complications, such as PJK and rod failure.[25]

SUMMARY

Pedicle subtraction osteotomies are an outstanding tool in the treatment of adult spinal deformity. They are useful in revision surgery as well as in the treatment of severe, rigid curves. However, surgeons must be aware of the higher complication rates associated with osteotomies and should carefully review the lessons and newly derived technique modifications illustrated in the recent literature.

REFERENCES

1. Thomasen E. Vertebral osteotomy for correction of kyphosis in ankylosing spondylitis. Clin Orthop Relat Res 1985;194:142–52.
2. Bridwell KH, Lewis SJ, Lenke LG, et al. Pedicle subtraction osteotomy for the treatment of fixed sagittal imbalance. J Bone Joint Surg Am 2003; 85-A:454–63.
3. Dorward IG, Lenke LG. Osteotomies in the posterior-only treatment of complex adult spinal deformity: a comparative review. Neurosurg Focus 2010;28:E4.
4. La Marca F, Brumblay H. Smith-Petersen osteotomy in thoracolumbar deformity surgery. Neurosurgery 2008;63:163–70.
5. Auerbach JD, Lenke LG, Bridwell KH, et al. Major complications and comparison between 3-column osteotomy techniques in 105 consecutive spinal deformity procedures. Spine (Phila Pa 1976) 2012; 37:1198–210.
6. Smith JS, Shaffrey CI, Ames CP, et al. Assessment of symptomatic rod fracture after posterior instrumented fusion for adult spinal deformity. Neurosurgery 2012;71:862–7.
7. Gupta S, Eksi MS, Ames CP, et al. A novel 4-rod technique offers potential to reduce rod breakage and pseudoarthrosis in pedicle subtraction osteotomies for adult spinal deformity correction. Oper Neurosurg (Hagerstown) 2017. https://doi.org/10.1093/ons/opx151.
8. Berjano P, Aebi M. Pedicle subtraction osteotomies (PSO) in the lumbar spine for sagittal deformities. Eur Spine J 2015;24(Suppl 1):S49–57.
9. Anderson AL, McIff TE, Asher MA, et al. The effect of posterior thoracic spine anatomical structures on motion segment flexion stiffness. Spine (Phila Pa 1976) 2009;34:441–6.
10. Wang Y, Zhang ÆY, Zhang ÆX, et al. A single posterior approach for multilevel modified vertebral column resection in adults with severe rigid congenital kyphoscoliosis: a retrospective study of 13 cases. Eur Spine J 2008;17(3):361–72.
11. Osteotomy PS, Wang H, Ma L, et al. Comparison of clinical and radiological improvement between the modified trephine and high-speed drill as main osteotomy instrument in pedicle subtraction osteotomy. Medicine (Baltimore) 2015;94(45): e2027.

12. Voyadzis JM, Gala VC, O'Toole JE, et al. Minimally invasive posterior osteotomies. Neurosurgery 2008; 63(3 Suppl):204–10.

13. Elgafy H, Bransford RJ, McGuire RA, et al. Blood loss in major spine surgery: are there effective measures to decrease massive hemorrhage in major spine fusion surgery? Spine (Phila Pa 1976) 2010; 35(9 Suppl):S47–56.

14. Buchowski JM, Bridwell KH, Lenke LG, et al. Neurologic complications of lumbar pedicle subtraction osteotomy a 10-year assessment. Spine (Phila Pa 1976) 2007;32:2245–52.

15. Theologis AA, Tabaraee E, Funao H, et al. Three-column osteotomies of the lower cervical and upper thoracic spine: comparison of early outcomes, radiographic parameters, and peri-operative complications in 48 patients. Eur Spine J 2014;24:23–30.

16. McMaster MJ. Osteotomy of the cervical spine in ankylosing spondylitis. J Bone Joint Surg Br 1997; 79:197–203.

17. Smith JS, Shaffrey E, Klineberg E, et al. Prospective multicenter assessment of risk factors for rod fracture following surgery for adult spinal deformity. J Neurosurg Spine 2014;21:994–1003.

18. Hallager DW, Karstensen S, Bukhari N, et al. Radiographic predictors for mechanical failure after adult spinal deformity surgery. Spine (Phila Pa 1976) 2017;42:E855–63.

19. Kim YJ, Bridwell KH, Lenke LG, et al. Pseudoarthrosis in long adult spinal deformity instrumentation and fusion to the sacrum: prevalence and risk factor analysis of 144 cases. Spine (Phila Pa 1976) 2006;31:2329–36.

20. Hyun SJ, Lenke LG, Kim YC, et al. Comparison of standard 2-rod constructs to multiple-rod constructs for fixation across 3-column spinal osteotomies. Spine (Phila Pa 1976) 2014;39:1899–904.

21. Hallager DW, Gehrchen M, Dahl B, et al. Use of supplemental short pre-contoured accessory rods and cobalt chrome alloy posterior rods reduces primary rod strain and range of motion across the pedicle subtraction osteotomy level: an in vitro biomechanical study. Spine (Phila Pa 1976) 2016; 41:E388–95.

22. Luca A, Ottardi C, Sasso M, et al. Instrumentation failure following pedicle subtraction osteotomy: the role of rod material, diameter, and multi-rod constructs. Eur Spine J 2017;26:764–70.

23. Tang JA, Leasure JM, Smith JS, et al. Effect of severity of rod contour on posterior rod failure in the setting of lumbar pedicle subtraction osteotomy (PSO): a biomechanical study. Neurosurgery 2013; 72:276–83.

24. Lafage V, Schwab FJ, Vira S, et al. Does vertebral level of pedicle subtraction osteotomy correlate with degree of spinopelvic parameter correction? J Neurosurg Spine 2011;14:184–91.

25. Yilgor C, Sogunmez N, Boissiere L, et al. Global alignment and proportion (GAP) score. J Bone Jt Surg 2017;99:1661–72.

Preventing Pseudoarthrosis and Proximal Junctional Kyphosis
How to Deal with the Osteoporotic Spine

Isaac O. Karikari, MD[a],*, Lionel N. Metz, MD[b]

KEYWORDS

- Spine fusion • Pseudoarthrosis • Nonunion • Osteoporosis • Proximal junctional kyphosis
- Screw failure • Compression fracture

KEY POINTS

- Patients with osteoporosis have a higher incidence of instrumentation-related complications.
- Preoperative optimization of bone quality is vital to ensure successful surgical outcome.
- Several intraoperative techniques exist to deal with some of the challenges that exist with the osteoporotic spine.

INTRODUCTION

Osteoporosis is a bony structural disorder characterized by discontinuity and thinning of the bony trabeculae leading to a decrease in the bone density despite a relatively normal biochemical composition.[1] Osteoporosis is defined by the World Health Organization as a T-score of less than 2.5, which represents a bone mineral density (BMD) 2.5 standard deviations less than the BMD of the average 25 year old.[2] There are 3 types of osteoporosis. Type I (postmenopausal) is encountered in women between 50 and 60 years of age due to low estrogen levels and in men with hypogonadic men. Type II (senile) is observed in men and women older than 70 years. Type III (secondary) osteoporosis occurs as a result of medical conditions or as side effects of medications, such as steroids.[3] The incidence of osteoporosis in patients undergoing spine surgery who are older than 50 years is reported to be 14.5% of men and 51.3% of women[4] (Fig. 1). Elderly patients with osteoporosis demonstrate an overall decrease in osteoblastic activity, poor vascularity, and limited functional bone marrow, which leads to less dense bone and a compromised capacity for bone healing and regeneration. Patients with osteoporosis exhibit defective osteogenic, osteoinductive, and osteoconductive abilities, which negatively impacts bone remodeling and fusion rates.[5] By virtue of exhibiting decreased pullout strength, cutout torque, and insertional torque, osteoporotic patients undergoing spine instrumentation are at a substantial risk of developing vertebral fractures, pseudoarthrosis, and instrumentation failure[6–10] (Fig. 2). It is, therefore, imperative for patients undergoing spinal instrumentation to undergo the appropriate screening and treatment before surgical intervention. The purpose of this article is to detail the optimal management of patients with degenerative lumbar deformity and osteoporosis, including preoperative preparation, intraoperative surgical strategies, and postoperative care.

Disclosure Statement: N/A.
a Department of Neurosurgery, Duke University Medical Center, 200 Trent Drive, Box 3807, Durham, NC 27710, USA; b Department of Orthopedic Surgery, University of California San Francisco, 500 Parnassus Avenue, MU-320-West, San Francisco, CA 94143, USA
* Corresponding author.
E-mail address: Isaac.karikari@duke.edu

Neurosurg Clin N Am 29 (2018) 365–374
https://doi.org/10.1016/j.nec.2018.03.005
1042-3680/18/© 2018 Elsevier Inc. All rights reserved.

neurosurgery.theclinics.com

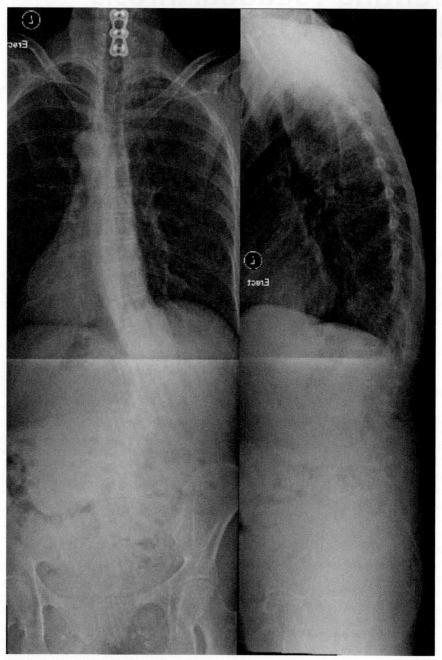

Fig. 1. Preoperative anteroposterior/lateral erect radiographs depicting poor bone quality in a 52-year-old woman with adult degenerative scoliosis. The presence of osteoporotic bone makes it difficult to visualize the spinal bony anatomy.

Preoperative Medical Treatments

It is recommended that asymptomatic women older than 65 years and men older than 70 years undergoing consideration for spinal fusion undergo screening for osteoporosis.[11] In addition, osteoporosis screening is recommended for at-risk younger patients, such as women with estrogen deficiency, low body mass, cigarette smoking, and prior history of compressive fracture. Once diagnosed with osteopenia or osteoporosis, several treatment modalities exist to optimize bone quality in preparation for surgery.[11]

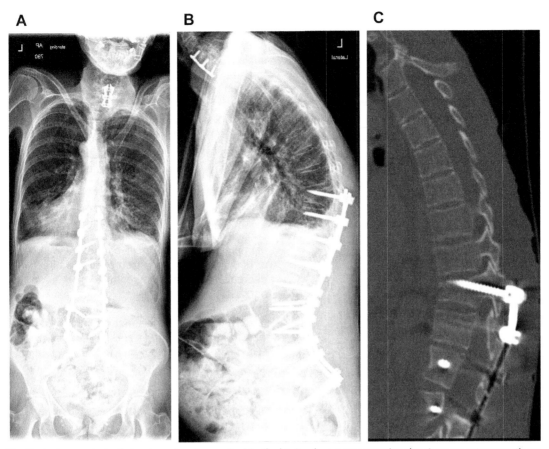

Fig. 2. Anteroposterior/lateral erect radiographs (*A, B*) obtained on postoperative day 4 on an osteoporotic patient, which demonstrate early mild compression deformity with evidence of early proximal junctional kyphosis. (*C*) Wedge compression fracture with fracture widening of the pedicle.

First, oral vitamin supplementation with calcium alone or in combination with vitamin D has been shown to prevent bone loss and fragility fractures.[12] Pharmacologic treatment of osteoporosis includes the use of bisphosphonates (eg, pamidronate, ibandronate, etidronate, and alendronate) and parathyroid hormone (PTH). Bisphosphonates function by promoting apoptosis of osteoclasts, which attenuates bone remodeling and reduces the risk of fracture and accelerated bone loss in patients with osteoporosis but does not contribute to new bone formation or remodeling. In a randomized control trial of 40 osteoporotic patients undergoing posterior lumbar interbody fusion, bisphosphonate treatment led to a significant increase in fusion rate at 1 year (95% vs 65% in the alendronate and control groups, respectively).[13] PTH is a hormone that works as an anabolic agent when dosed with temporal pulsing. PTH works by promoting increased bone formation by preventing apoptosis of osteoblasts.[14–17] Recombinant PTH commercialized as teriparatide binds to a G protein–coupled, PTH-related peptide receptor on osteoblast, which activates a downstream signaling pathway leading to increased intracellular calcium and gene expression of bone-forming growth factors.[18] Teriparatide is administered as a once-daily subcutaneous injection, reaching maximum serum concentration in 30 minutes. The bioavailability of teriparatide is 95%, and the half-life is approximately 1 hour.[18] Although teriparatide is more expensive, its clinical effectiveness over other osteoporotic therapies is unequivocal. This finding was suggested in a prospective trial in which 57 women with osteoporosis and degenerative spondylolisthesis undergoing posterolateral fusion were treated with either PTH or bisphosphonate. The rate of bone union was 82% in the PTH group and 68% in the bisphosphonate group.[19]

In patients with estrogen deficiency, such as elderly postmenopausal women, estrogen and selective estrogen receptor modulators have been shown to be effective in improving bone quality and enhancing spinal fusion.[20–22] This class of medications functions by stimulating an estrogenic response in bone tissue thereby stimulating osteoblast to increase bone formation.[20–22]

Lastly, calcitonin that is administered intranasally and works by directly inhibiting the function of osteoclast has been shown to reduce the risks of spinal fractures by 33% compared with placebo in a randomized control trial.[23,24]

Intraoperative Considerations for Osteoporotic Patients

Despite medical optimization in patients with osteoporosis undergoing spinal fusion surgery, intraoperative decisions and techniques play a vital role in the overall radiographic and clinical outcomes of patients with poor bone quality. There is a plethora of techniques that have been recommended to help mitigate some of challenges faced with the osteoporotic bone.

The use of large-diameter, long pedicle screws at multiple fixation points is an effective strategy in long fusion constructs.[25,26] Larger-diameter screws structurally fill more of the pedicle thereby engaging the stronger pedicle cortex, which minimizes the screw toggle within the pedicle. Longer pedicle screws allow more threads in bone and in vertebral levels like the sacrum allow for engagement of the ventral cortex.[25–29] The S1 screw placed in a tricortical trajectory aiming for the sacral promontory engages posterior, anterior, and anterosuperior cortices, which have been demonstrated to increase the insertional torque of an S1 screw placed in such a position[30] (**Fig. 3**). Placement of a cortical screw trajectory has been shown to increase insertional torque and the pullout strength of screws. The cortical screw trajectory travels in a dorsomedial to ventrolateral trajectory, which effectively engages more

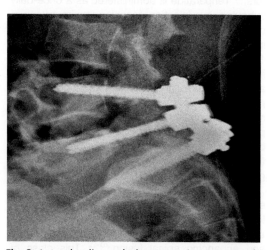

Fig. 3. Lateral radiograph demonstrating an example of a tricortical screw. The screw that is aimed for the sacral promontory engages posterior, anterior, and anterosuperior cortices of the sacrum.

screw threads in the cortical bone in the pars interarticularis and the pedicle.[31–34]

Reinforcement of screws with the addition of sublaminar wires or lamina hooks can accentuate the strength of fixation by increasing the pullout strength, stiffness, and torsional stability in osteoporotic bone.[35–38]

The use of expanded screw designs has been shown to improve fixation strength by increasing the pullout residence by 50% in one study.[39–41] The screw works by compressing the cancellous bone within the vertebral body as they expand, which increases the density of bone around the screw.[39]

The screw insertion technique is an important consideration in the osteoporotic spine. The diameter of the pilot hole cannot be oversized or undersized. An oversized pilot hole effectively decreases the screw purchase, whereas an undersized pilot hole, although increasing the insertional torque, may lead to pedicle fracture.[42] The optimal diameter of the pilot hole was studied by Battula and colleagues,[42] who investigated the pullout strength and insertional torque of self-tapping screws in osteoporotic bone. The investigators found that creating a pilot hole no larger than 71.5% of the outer diameter of the screw minimizes pullout and iatrogenic fracture.[42]

The positive impact of undertapping of the pedicle screw tracks has been extensively studied.[7,43] Kuklo and colleagues,[43] in a cadaveric studied, reported an increased insertional torque by 47% and 93% in osteoporotic vertebrae when the pedicle was undertapped by 0.5 and 1.0 mm, respectively. Similarly, Halvorson and colleagues[7] found that not tapping or undertapping the pedicle screw by 1 mm resulted in a significantly stronger screw pullout strength than tapping to the same size as the inserted pedicle.

Cement augmentation is an effective consideration in patients undergoing complex spinal fusions. The addition of cement mantle around a pedicle screw improves fixation of the screw and distributes stresses in the adjacent trabeculae thereby decreasing the tendency for screw loosening and pullout[44,45] (**Fig. 4**).

Strategies to Reduce Pseudoarthrosis in the Osteoporotic Spine

Osteoporotic patients undergoing a spinal fusion surgery are faced with a significant challenge in the race between loss of fixation and achievement of solid fusion. The achievement of rapid solid bony fusion is critical, as time is of the essence in this patient population. Prevention of

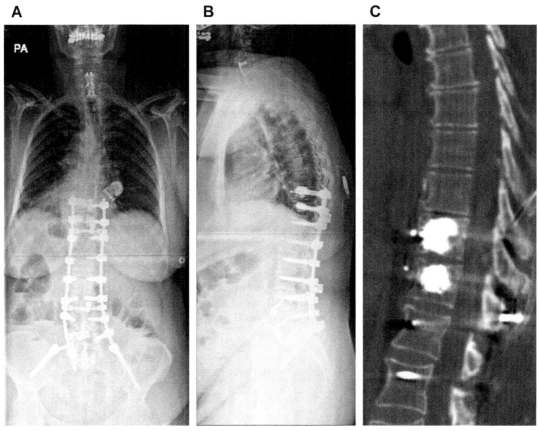

Fig. 4. (A) Anteroposterior and (B) lateral radiographs and (C) sagittal CT image of a patient with poor bone quality undergoing a multilevel fusion. Cement augmentation is used at the upper instrumented level (T10) and T11 to increase screw purchase and pullout strength.

pseudoarthrosis begins with preoperative optimization of risks factors. Among the factors that have been associated with an increased rate of pseudoarthrosis and must be optimized include nicotine use, vitamin D deficiency, diabetes mellitus, alcoholism, and osteoporosis.[46]

Intraoperatively, the achievement of spinopelvic balance is an important goal in the surgical management of lumbar degenerative deformity. Positive sagittal alignment biomechanically places excessive stress/strain on posterior instrumentation and fusion mass and contributes to instrumentation failure and pseudoarthrosis. In a retrospective review of 144 adult patients undergoing spinal deformity surgery, Kim and colleagues reported positive sagittal balance as a significant risk factor for the development of pseudoarthrosis. Further, the creation of a good surface area with decortication and adequate bone grafting with rich vascular supply are prerequisites for the formation of a solid fusion mass.[47] The choice of bone graft material used plays a significant role in the creation of a solid fusion mass. Although several bone graft materials exist, autogenous iliac crest bone is considered the gold standard because of

its osteogenic, osteoinductive, and osteoconductive properties. However, iliac crest bone has a limited supply; iliac bone graft harvesting has been associated with increased donor site morbidity, increased operative time, and blood loss.[48] This increased morbidity served as an impetus for the search for efficacious bone graft alternatives, including allograft materials and synthetic materials. Bone morphogenic proteins are the auto-inductive factor in bone, and recombinant human bone morphogenetic protein-2 (rhBMP-2, INFUSE, Medtronic Sofamor Danek, Memphis, TN) is a potent osteo-biological device to induce spinal fusion. rhBMP-2 was approved by the Food and Drug Administration (FDA) for anterior lumbar interbody fusion (ALIF) in 2002. Although rhBMP-2 was FDA approved for ALIF, off-label use in posterior fusions in high risks cases (eg, osteoporosis) is common. A prospective study by Mulconrey and colleagues[49] reported excellent fusion rates using rhBMP-2 in patients undergoing multilevel adult spinal deformity surgery obviating iliac crest bone graft. Superiority of rhBMP-2 has been suggested in some human studies.[50,51] Dimar and colleagues[50] performed a prospective randomized study comparing rhBMP-2 with iliac crest graft for single level posterolateral lumbar fusion in which they reported a 91% fusion rate in the rhBMP-2 group compared with 73% in the group receiving the iliac crest graft. Similarly, Kim and colleagues[51] reported a superior fusion rate in patients undergoing adult spinal deformity surgery with rhBMP-2 compared with iliac crest graft. In their study, patients receiving rhBMP-2 achieved a 93.5% fusion rate compared with 71.9% in the iliac crest graft group. The use of rhBMP-2 is not without side effects, however. Complications reported include bone resorption/osteolysis, heterotopic/ectopic bone formation, radiculitis, wound infection, seroma formation, and cancer.[52–58]

Postoperatively, the failure of instrumentation in osteoporotic patients usually occurs through screw toggling, loosening, and eventual pullout (see **Fig. 1**). The mainstay strategy in managing early postoperative instrumentation-related complications in osteoporotic patients consists of brace therapy, continuation of medical therapies for osteoporosis, and prevention of falls. The optimal duration of brace therapy and type of brace are not currently well established.

Strategies to Reduce Proximal Junctional Kyphosis in Osteoporotic Patients

Proximal junctional kyphosis (PJK) is the progressive flexion (kyphosis) of adjacent segments proximal to a long spinal fusion. PJK may be the result of any combination of the following causes: failure of the posterior tension band due to soft tissue disruption or attenuation, in particular the supraspinous and interspinous ligaments, para-spinous muscle dysfunction, or facet joint disruption; intervertebral disk degeneration; instrumentation failure; and/or compression fracture of the upper instrumented vertebra (UIV) or the supra-adjacent vertebra.[59] Often PJK can be asymptomatic and be treated with observation. Operative treatment may be indicated in cases whereby kyphosis is progressive or accompanied by significant pain or a neurologic deficit.[60]

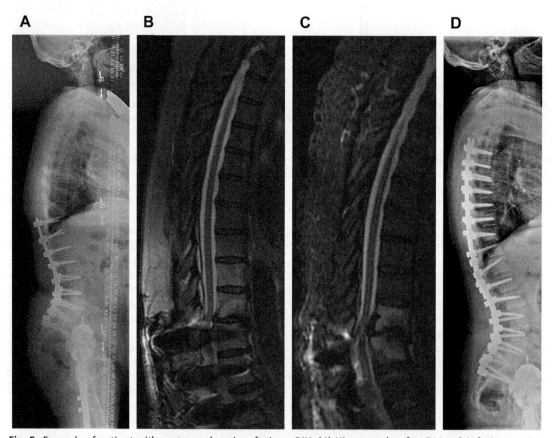

Fig. 5. Example of patient with acute on chronic soft tissue PJK. (*A*) Nine months after T11-pelvis fusion routine imaging shows PJK; patient has pain but no neurologic deficit. (*B*) MRI 11 months postoperative shows stenosis; patient has not deficits. (*C*) Patient has fall and presents with new bilateral lower extremity weakness; large disk extrusion present on MRI. (*D*) Extension of fusion to T4, laminectomy/discectomy, and type 2 osteotomy with transforaminal thoracic interbody fusion placed. Patient recovered to baseline strength within 3 months.

Lee and Park[59] reported an incidence of junctional kyphosis after multilevel fusion in a range between 6% and 41% in their literature review. Kim and colleagues[61] demonstrated a rate of 17% to 39% in as systematic review of 8 studies characterizing PJK in patients with deformity. Ha and colleagues[62] demonstrated a rate of radiographic PJK of 34% for fusions to the thoracolumbar junction and 27% for patients with an upper thoracic UIV in a single-institution study. Furthermore, the group found that compression fracture at the UIV was more prevalent in the thoracolumbar group, whereas subluxation was more prevalent in the proximal thoracic group. Nine percent of the thoracolumbar PJK group required further surgery, whereas 12% in the proximal thoracic required revision. This study also found that the onset of PJK requiring surgery was significantly earlier in thoracolumbar group, usually occurring within the first year.

Given the finding that most cases of thoracolumbar PJK involved compression fracture,

osteoporosis is a particularly potent risk factor for PJK with a thoracolumbar UIV; therefore, preoperative optimization of bone density is highly recommended.

Soft tissue disruption is a detrimental side effect of instrumentation and may contribute to PJK. Ligament restoration and augmentation strategies have been used to mitigate this factor. Zaghloul and colleagues[63] recorded no cases of PJK in their first 18 patients who underwent Mersilene strap stabilization of the supra-adjacent spinous processes in a cohort of patients with primary and revision deformity. Safaee and colleagues[64] have also shown promising results in preventing PJK in high-risk patients by using a combination approach of vertebroplasty, transverse process hooks, terminal rod contouring, and ligament augmentation using sublaminar cables passed through the supra-adjacent spinous processes and affixed to the terminal end of the rods.

Symptomatic PJK is often diagnosed when patients return for follow-up with unremitting pain at

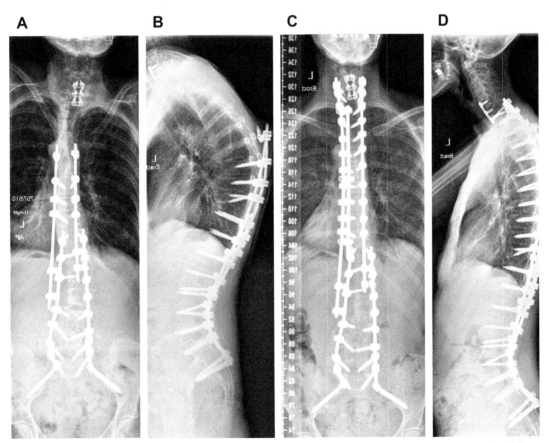

Fig. 6. Example of revision surgery following instrumentation failure in a patient with poor bone quality. (*A*) Preoperative anteroposterior (AP) radiographs. (*B*) Preoperative lateral radiographs demonstrating failure of instrumentation at the bone/implant interface with pullout of proximal hooks. (*C, D*) Postoperative (1 year) AP and lateral radiograph showing extension of instrumentation to C7 at the level of a previous anterior fusion. The presence of anterior fusion will help provide additional stability and reduce the flexion bending moment.

the top of the construct or more rarely neurologic deficit particularly in cases of severe kyphosis or subluxation[60] (**Fig. 5**). However, routine follow-up radiographs should be made at predetermined intervals to diagnose asymptomatic radiographic proximal kyphosis, as those patients may require closer follow-up. Cross-sectional imaging with MRI or CT myelogram to evaluate canal compromise and stenosis is imperative, as shown in **Fig. 5**. A CT scan to document screw purchase and healing of previous arthrodesis levels can help finalize an operative plan. The CT scan or a supine lateral radiograph will also allow the surgeon to understand the reducibility of the deformity and plan surgical treatment accordingly. Depending on the severity of the kyphosis and the rigidity of the deformity, treatment may involve extension of fusion only or the use of on osteotomy (type II through type VI)[65] to restore normal sagittal alignment.[66] When extension of fusion is required for pseudoarthrosis/PJK, the addition of anterior support in the revision surgery helps reduce flexion-bending force on the posterior instrumentation in addition to enhancing fusion rates[67,68] (**Fig. 6**).

Osteoporosis is an important comorbidity in patients with degenerative lumbar deformity. Preoperative identification and treatment of osteoporosis, intraoperative strategies to improve fixation, and postoperative pharmacologic treatment and protection are useful strategies for the optimal management of patients with osteoporosis and spinal deformity.

REFERENCES

1. Hart RA, Prendergast MA. Spine surgery for lumbar degenerative disease in elderly and osteoporotic patients. Instr Course Lect 2007;56:257–72.

2. WHO Scientific Group. Prevention and management of osteoporosis. World Health Organ Tech Rep Ser 2003;921:1–164.

3. Dodwad SM, Khan SN. Surgical stabilization of the spine in the osteoporotic patient. Orthop Clin North Am 2013;44(2):243–9.

4. Chin DK, Park JY, Yoon YS, et al. Prevalence of osteoporosis in patients requiring spine surgery: incidence and significance of osteoporosis in spine disease. Osteoporos Int 2007;18(9):1219–24.

5. Park SB, Chung CK. Strategies of spinal fusion on osteoporotic spine. J Korean Neurosurg Soc 2011; 49(6):317–22.

6. Wittenberg RH, Shea M, Swartz DE, et al. Importance of bone mineral density in instrumented spine fusions. Spine (Phila Pa 1976) 1991;16(6):647–52.

7. Halvorson TL, Kelley LA, Thomas KA, et al. Effects of bone mineral density on pedicle screw fixation. Spine (Phila Pa 1976) 1994;19(21):2415–20.

8. Okuyama K, Sato K, Abe E, et al. Stability of transpedicle screwing for the osteoporotic spine. An in vitro study of the mechanical stability. Spine (Phila Pa 1976) 1993;18(15):2240–5.

9. Paxinos O, Tsitsopoulos PP, Zindrick MR, et al. Evaluation of pullout strength and failure mechanism of posterior instrumentation in normal and osteopenic thoracic vertebrae. J Neurosurg Spine 2010;13(4): 469–76.

10. DeWald CJ, Stanley T. Instrumentation-related complications of multilevel fusions for adult spinal deformity patients over age 65: surgical considerations and treatment options in patients with poor bone quality. Spine (Phila Pa 1976) 2006;31(19 suppl):S144–51.

11. American College of Radiology. ACR-SPR-SSR practice parameter for the performance of dual-energy x-ray absorptiometry (DXA)—Res 31. Amended 2014 (Res 39, 2013). Available at: http://www.acr.org/_/media/ACR/Documents/PGTS/guidelines/DXA.pdf. Accessed December 1, 2018.

12. Gehrig L, Lane J, O'Connor MI. Osteoporosis: management and treatment strategies for orthopaedic surgeons. J Bone Joint Surg Am 2008;90(6):1362–74.

13. Nagahama K, Kanayama M, Togawa D, et al. Does alendronate disturb the healing process of posterior lumbar interbody fusion? A prospective randomized trial. J Neurosurg Spine 2011;14(4):500–7.

14. Roux S. New treatment targets in osteoporosis. Joint Bone Spine 2010;77(3):222–8.

15. Jilka RL, Weinstein RS, Bellido T, et al. Increased bone formation by prevention of osteoblast apoptosis with parathyroid hormone. J Clin Invest 1999;104(4):439–46.

16. Hughes DE, Wright KR, Uy HL, et al. Bisphosphonates promote apoptosis in murine osteoclasts in vitro and in vivo. J Bone Miner Res 1995;10(10):1478–87.

17. Hodsman AB, Bauer DC, Dempster DW, et al. Parathyroid hormone and teriparatide for the treatment of osteoporosis: a review of the evidence and suggested guidelines for its use. Endocr Rev 2005; 26(5):688–703.

18. Kraenzlin ME, Meier C. Parathyroid hormone analogues in the treatment of osteoporosis. Nat Rev Endocrinol 2011;7(11):647–56.

19. Ohtori S, Inoue G, Orita S, et al. Teriparatide accelerates lumbar posterolateral fusion in women with postmenopausal osteoporosis: prospective study. Spine (Phila Pa 1976) 2012;37(23):E1464–8.

20. Gardner MJ, Demetrakopoulos D, Shindle MK, et al. Osteoporosis and skeletal fractures. HSS J 2006; 2(1):62–9.

21. Ettinger B, Black DM, Mitlak BH, et al. Reduction of vertebral fracture risk in postmenopausal women with osteoporosis treated with raloxifene: results from a 3-year randomized clinical trial. Multiple Outcomes of Raloxifene Evaluation (MORE) investigators. JAMA 1999;282(7):637–45.

22. Sarkar S, Mitlak BH, Wong M, et al. Relationships between bone mineral density and incident vertebral fracture risk with raloxifene therapy. J Bone Miner Res 2002;17(1):1–10.

23. Chesnut CH, Silverman S, Andriano K, et al. A randomized trial of nasal spray salmon calcitonin in postmenopausal women with established osteoporosis: the prevent recurrence of osteoporotic fractures study. PROOF study group. Am J Med 2000; 109(4):267–76.

24. Lane JM, Gardner MJ, Lin JT, et al. The aging spine: new technologies and therapeutics for the osteoporotic spine. Eur Spine J 2003;12(suppl 2): S147–54.

25. Zindrick MR, Wiltse LL, Widell EH, et al. A biomechanical study of intrapeduncular screw fixation in the lumbosacral spine. Clin Orthop Relat Res 1986;(203):99–112.

26. Kwok AW, Finkelstein JA, Woodside T, et al. Insertional torque and pull-out strengths of conical and cylindrical pedicle screws in cadaveric bone. Spine (Phila Pa 1976) 1996;21(21):2429–34.

27. Tsai KJ, Murakami H, Horton WC, et al. Pedicle screw fixation strength: a biomechanical comparison between 4.5-mm and 5.5-mm diameter screws in osteoporotic upper thoracic vertebrae. J Surg Orthop Adv 2009;18(1):23–7.

28. Bianco RJ, Arnoux PJ, Wagnac E, et al. Minimizing pedicle screw pullout risks: a detailed biomechanical analysis of screw design and placement. Clin Spine Surg 2017;30(3):E226–32.

29. Brantley AG, Mayfield JK, Koeneman JB, et al. The effects of pedicle screw fit. An in vitro study. Spine (Phila Pa 1976) 1994;19(15):1752–8.

30. Lehman RA Jr, Kuklo TR, Belmont PJ Jr, et al. Advantage of pedicle screw fixation directed into the apex of the sacral promontory over bicortical fixation: a biomechanical analysis. Spine (Phila Pa 1976) 2002;27(8):806–11.

31. Santoni BG, Hynes RA, McGilvray KC, et al. Cortical bone trajectory for lumbar pedicle screws. Spine J 2009;9(5):366–73.

32. Wray S, Mimran R, Vadapalli S, et al. Pedicle screw placement in the lumbar spine: effect of trajectory and screw design on acute biomechanical purchase. J Neurosurg Spine 2015;22(5):1–8.

33. Matsukawa K, Yato Y, Nemoto O, et al. Morphometric measurement of cortical bone trajectory for lumbar pedicle screw insertion using computed tomography. J Spinal Disord Tech 2013;26(6): E248–53.

34. Inceoglu S, Montgomery WH Jr, St Clair S, et al. Pedicle screw insertion angle and pullout strength: comparison of 2 proposed strategies. J Neurosurg Spine 2011;14(5):670–6.

35. Coe JD, Warden KE, Herzig MA, et al. Influence of bone mineral density on the fixation of thoracolumbar implants. A comparative study of transpedicular screws, laminar hooks, and spinous process wires. Spine 1990;15:902–7.

36. Hasegawa K, Takahashi HE, Uchiyama S, et al. An experimental study of a combination method using a pedicle screw and laminar hook for the osteoporotic spine. Spine 1997;22:958–62.

37. Margulies JY, Casar RS, Caruso SA, et al. The mechanical role of laminar hook protection of pedicle screws at the caudal end vertebra. Eur Spine J 1997;6:245–8.

38. Tan JS, Kwon BK, Dvorak MF, et al. Pedicle screw motion in the osteoporotic spine after augmentation with laminar hooks, sublaminar wires, or calcium phosphate cement: a comparative analysis. Spine 2004;29:1723–30.

39. Cook SD, Salkeld SL, Whitecloud TS III, et al. Biomechanical evaluation and preliminary clinical experience with an expansive pedicle screw design. J Spinal Disord 2000;13(3):230–6.

40. Gao M, Lei W, Wu Z, et al. Biomechanical evaluation of fixation strength of conventional and expansive pedicle screws with or without calcium based cement augmentation. Clin Biomech 2011;26(3): 238–44.

41. Wu ZX, Gong FT, Liu L, et al. A comparative study on screw loosening in osteoporotic lumbar spine fusion between expandable and conventional pedicle screws. Arch Orthop Trauma Surg 2012;132(4): 471–6.

42. Battula S, Schoenfeld AJ, Sahai V, et al. The effect of pilot hole size on the insertion torque and pullout strength of self-tapping cortical bone screws in osteoporotic bone. J Trauma 2008; 64(4):990–5.

43. Kuklo TR, Lehman RA Jr. Effect of various tapping diameters on insertion of thoracic pedicle screws: a biomechanical analysis. Spine (Phila Pa 1976) 2003;28(18):2066–71.

44. Pfeifer BA, Krag MH, Johnson C. Repair of failed transpedicle screw fixation. A biomechanical study comparing polymethylmethacrylate, milled bone, and matchstick bone reconstruction. Spine (Phila Pa 1976) 1994;19(3):350–3.

45. Aydogan M, Ozturk C, Karatoprak O, et al. The pedicle screw fixation with vertebroplasty augmentation in the surgical treatment of the severe osteoporotic spines. J Spinal Disord Tech 2009;22(6): 444–7.

46. Rothman RH, Booth R. Failures of spinal fusion. Orthop Clin North Am 1975;6:299–304.

47. Steinmann JC, Herkowitz HN. Pseudoarthrosis of the spine. Clin Orthop Relat Res 1992;284:80–90.

48. Gruskay JA, Basques BA, Bohl DD, et al. Short-term adverse events, length of stay, and readmission after iliac crest bone graft for spinal fusion. Spine 2014;39(20):1718–24.

49. Mulconrey DS, Bridwell KH, Flynn J, et al. Bone morphogenetic protein (rhBMP-2) as a substitute for iliac crest bone graft in multilevel adult spinal deformity surgery: minimum two-year evaluation of fusion. Spine 2008;33(20):2153–9.

50. Dimar JR, Glassman SD, Burkus KJ, et al. Clinical outcomes and fusion success at 2 years of single-level instrumented posterolateral fusions with recombinant human bone morphogenetic protein-2/compression resistant matrix versus iliac crest bone graft. Spine 2006;31:2534–9.

51. Kim HJ, Buchowski JM, Zebala LP, et al. RhBMP-2 is superior to iliac crest bone graft for long fusions to the sacrum in adult spinal deformity: 4- to 14-year follow-up. Spine 2013;38(14):1209–15.

52. Lewandrowski KU, Nanson C, Calderon R. Vertebral osteolysis after posterior interbody lumbar fusion with recombinant human bone morphogenetic protein 2: a report of five cases. Spine J 2007;7(5):609–14.

53. Pradhan BB, Bae HW, Dawson EG, et al. Graft resorption with the use of bone morphogenetic protein: lessons from anterior lumbar interbody fusion using femoral ring allografts and recombinant human bone morphogenetic protein-2. Spine 2006;31:E277–84.

54. Sandhu HS, Toth JM, Diwan AD, et al. Histologic evaluation of the efficacy of rhBMP-2 compared with autograft bone in sheep spinal anterior interbody fusion. Spine 2002;27:567–75.

55. Tannoury CA, An HS. Complications with the use of bone morphogenetic protein 2 (BMP-2) in spine surgery. Spine J 2014;14(3):552–9.

56. Chrastil J, Low JB, Whang PG, et al. Complications associated with the use of the recombinant human bone morphogenetic proteins for posterior interbody fusions of the lumbar spine. Spine 2013;38(16):E1020–7.

57. Joseph V, Rampersaud YR. Heterotopic bone formation with the use of rhBMP2 in posterior minimal access interbody fusion: a CT analysis. Spine 2007;32(25):2885–90.

58. Mindea SA, Shih P, Song JK. Recombinant human bone morphogenetic protein-2-induced radiculitis in elective minimally invasive transforaminal lumbar interbody fusions: a series review. Spine 2009;34(14):1480–4.

59. Lee J, Park YS. Proximal junctional kyphosis: diagnosis, pathogenesis, and treatment. Asian Spine J 2016;10:593–600.

60. Watanabe K, Lenke LG, Bridwell KH, et al. Proximal junctional vertebral fracture in adults after spinal deformity surgery using pedicle screw constructs: analysis of morphological features. Spine (Phila Pa 1976) 2010;35:138–45.

61. Kim HJ, Lenke LG, Shaffrey CI, et al. Proximal junctional kyphosis as a distinct form of adjacent segment pathology after spinal deformity surgery: a systematic review. Spine (Phila Pa 1976) 2012;37:S144–64.

62. Ha Y, Maruo K, Racine L, et al. Proximal junctional kyphosis and clinical outcomes in adult spinal deformity surgery with fusion from the thoracic spine to the sacrum: a comparison of proximal and distal upper instrumented vertebrae. J Neurosurg Spine 2013;19:360–9.

63. Zaghloul KM, Matoian BJ, Denardin NB, et al. Preventing proximal adjacent level kyphosis with strap stabilization. Orthopedics 2016;39:794–9.

64. Safaee MM, Osorio JA, Verma K, et al. Proximal junctional kyphosis prevention strategies: a video technique guide. Oper Neurosurg (Hagerstown) 2017;13:581–5.

65. Schwab F, Blondel B, Chay E, et al. The comprehensive anatomical spinal osteotomy classification. Neurosurgery 2014;74:112–20.

66. McClendon J, O'Shaughnessy BA, Sugrue PA, et al. Techniques for operative correction of proximal junctional kyphosis of the upper thoracic spine. Spine (Phila Pa 1976) 2012;37:292–303.

67. Lund T, Oxland TR, Jost B, et al. Interbody cage stabilization in the lumbar spine: biomechanical evaluation of cage design, posterior instrumentation and bone density. J Bone Joint Surg Br 1998;80:351–9.

68. McAfee PC. Interbody fusion cages in reconstructive operations on the spine. J Bone Joint Surg Am 1999;81:859–80.

The Challenge of Creating Lordosis in High-Grade Dysplastic Spondylolisthesis

Ryan J. Hoel, MD[a], Robert M. Brenner, MS, MD[a],
David W. Polly Jr, MD[a,b],*

KEYWORDS

- High-grade spondylolisthesis • Dysplastic spondylolisthesis • Spondyloptosis • Sagittal balance

KEY POINTS

- High-grade dysplastic spondylolisthesis (HGDS) is secondary to dysplastic lumbosacral morphology and frequently results in sagittal imbalance secondary to kyphosis of L5 relative to S1.
- Reduction at the time of fusion improves sagittal balance and decreases the rate of pseudarthrosis.
- As the lumbosacral kyphosis, rather than translation, drives the pelvis and spine into imbalance, the foremost focus in any reduction must be to restore lumbosacral lordosis.
- Most techniques for reduction achieve similar correction with similar complication rates.
- Recent literature demonstrates minimal difference in postoperative neurologic deficits in HGDS patients treated with reduction and fusion versus in situ fusion.

INTRODUCTION

Dysplastic spondylolisthesis is a subset of L5-S1 spondylolisthesis that occurs because of dysplastic lumbosacral anatomy. Prior works have shown that more severe dysplasia is associated with higher grades of spondylolisthesis, with those slips greater than 50% (Meyerding grades III, IV, and V) classified as "high grade."[1] Studies have shown that most patients with HGDS will develop pain and/or neural deficits over time if managed nonoperatively.[2] Surgical treatment of symptomatic high-grade spondylolisthesis is often appropriate to treat existing deformity and to prevent further progression of deformity. However, the optimal algorithm and technique remain controversial. The purpose of this article is to review the modern understanding of HGDS with respect to its effect on spinal sagittal alignment, to detail several techniques for obtaining sagittal correction intraoperatively, and to evaluate current evidence regarding surgical complications.

SAGITTAL ALIGNMENT IN HIGH-GRADE DYSPLASTIC SPONDYLOLISTHESIS

High-grade dysplastic spondylolisthesis (HGDS) results in significant deformity and compromise of the normal sagittal profile of the spine. Patients with HGDS have altered sacral and spinopelvic morphology with an increased pelvic incidence compared with the general population.[3] High-grade spondylolisthesis typically results in kyphosis of the L5 vertebra relative to S1. These

Disclosure Statement: No industry conflicts of interest. Dr D.W. Polly has been a clinical investigator in a clinical trial sponsored by SI-Bone, but has not received any financial remuneration. No funding was received for this work.

[a] Department of Orthopaedic Surgery, University of Minnesota, 2450 Riverside Avenue South, Suite R200, Minneapolis, MN 55454, USA; [b] Department of Neurosurgery, University of Minnesota, 2450 Riverside Avenue South, Suite R200, Minneapolis, MN 55454, USA

* Corresponding author. Department of Orthopaedic Surgery, University of Minnesota, 2450 Riverside Avenue South, Suite R200, Minneapolis, MN 55454.

E-mail address: pollydw@umn.edu

patients first compensate through increased intervertebral segmental lumbar lordosis (LL) leading to an overall increase in total LL. To further compensate for worsened focal L5-S1 kyphosis, increased LL is followed by increased pelvic retroversion, increasing the pelvic tilt (PT) while decreasing the sacral slope (SS). Once these 2 physiologic compensation mechanisms cannot adequately counteract the L5-S1 kyphosis, the patient acquires an overall positive sagittal imbalance, which is subsequently compensated for with hip flexion and knee flexion, caused by an extension block from hyperlordosis and a retroverted pelvis, leading to the Phalen-Dickson gait.[4]

Labelle and colleagues[4] in conjunction with the Spine Deformity Study Group developed a classification of L5-S1 spondylolisthesis, of which types 4, 5, and 6 reflect the overall pelvic and spinal balance of high-grade spondylolisthesis specifically (**Fig. 1**). Type 4 denotes an HGDS that is able to maintain a balanced pelvis; type 5 is a pelvis that has increased retroversion with maintenance of overall spinal sagittal alignment, and type 6 refers to an HGDS that has overcome the ability of LL and pelvic retroversion to adequately compensate, resulting in global spinal sagittal alignment.[4] The defining values of PT and SS demarcating a balanced or unbalanced pelvis were defined in a nomogram by Hresko and colleagues.[5] The spinal sagittal profile deteriorated from normalcy in the retroverted pelvic group, exhibiting greater L5 incidence, lumbosacral angle, length of LL, and less thoracic kyphosis than the balanced pelvic group.[5]

Harroud and colleagues[6] showed that worse global sagittal alignment parameters correlated with worse quality of life in nonoperatively managed HGDS patients, suggesting that global sagittal alignment should be critically evaluated in any HGDS patient. In addition, Blondel and colleagues[7] showed that the best health-related quality-of-life outcomes were achieved with near complete sagittal plane deformity correction, whereas patients with only modest correction achieved clinically insignificant improvement. Labelle classification types 5 and 6 represent those patients who may merit more aggressive attempts at reduction during surgery, because they are the result of the patient's inability to adequately compensate for the HGDS. Therefore, in HGDS with an unbalanced pelvis (types 5 and 6), it is the authors' preferred technique to perform reduction to best accomplish these goals.

Before this modern understanding of the effect of the lumbosacral kyphosis on overall sagittal alignment, much of the emphasis during reduction was focused on reducing the translational slip grade. Because the lumbosacral kyphosis, rather than translation, drives the pelvis and spine into imbalance, the foremost focus in any reduction must be to restore lumbosacral lordosis.

EVIDENCE FAVORING REDUCTION

Principal to the argument in favor of reduction is that the patient's sagittal parameters can be improved, as compared with an in situ fusion in which the sagittal malalignment is maintained. The authors' clinical experience has shown some patients with in situ fusions present decades later with severe global sagittal imbalance and pain, and subsequent surgical management is exceptionally challenging (**Fig. 2**). In addition, multiple studies have shown a lower rate of pseudarthrosis with reduction compared with in situ fusion. This finding was further borne out in a systematic review by Longo and colleagues,[8] who found a pseudarthrosis rate of 5.5% in HGDS patients treated with reduction, compared with 17.8% in those fused in situ. The explanation for this finding is that compared with an in situ fusion, a full or partial reduction of high-grade spondylolisthesis results in less shear at the lumbosacral junction and provides a better biomechanical environment for fusion.[9]

SURGICAL REDUCTION TECHNIQUES

Multiple techniques have been described to aid in the reduction of HGDS. Most contemporary studies have used an interbody fusion, with many

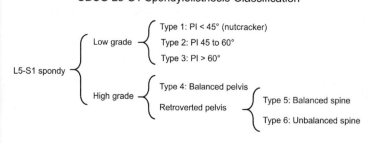

SDSG L5-S1 Spondylolisthesis Classification

Fig. 1. Classification of spondylolisthesis based on spinopelvic posture. PI, pelvic incidence. (*From* Labelle H, Mac-Thiong J-M, Roussouly P. Spinopelvic sagittal balance of spondylolisthesis: a review and classification. Eur Spine J 2011;20(S5):643; with permission.)

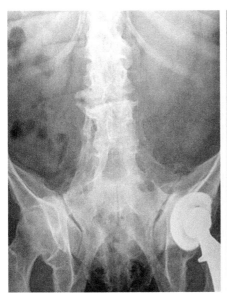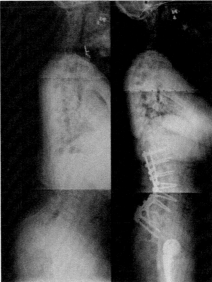

Fig. 2. Preoperative and postoperative images of a 42-year-old woman who presented with chronic pain due to sagittal imbalance after an in situ fusion had been performed several decades before, requiring extensive surgery to remove the fusion mass and restore LL.

investigators describing an all-posterior approach, performing a transforaminal interbody fusion (TLIF) at L5-S1. Descriptions of each reduction technique will be detailed in the following section. Details of the sagittal correction reported by investigators using these techniques can be found in **Table 1**.

External Reduction Measures

Closed reduction and casting of spondylolisthesis were described by Scaglietti and colleagues,[10] and Bradford and Boachie-Adjei[11] subsequently showed that a 3-stage procedure, including initial decompression, 10 days of skeletal traction, and subsequent anterior reduction and fusion, were efficacious in improvement of sagittal alignment. Notable drawbacks to these techniques are their time-intensive nature, requirement for prolonged inpatient treatments, and need for prolonged bed rest during the traction period. Because of the drawbacks, these techniques are now rarely performed.

External Transpedicular Fixation

Magerl[12] described a technique in which transpedicular Schanz pins are connected to an external apparatus capable of providing distraction and compression forces across the vertebrae. This technique was subsequently used by surgeons treating patients with HGDS as a method for reduction, who found that the technique reliably improved sagittal parameters.[13] Benefits of this

strategy over prolonged halo traction are the ability to ambulate while the fixator is in place, and the ability to monitor for neurologic changes as the reduction is slowly achieved. Drawbacks are a high rate of pin site complications (noted to be up to 33%), the burden of a posterior external fixator device preventing the supine position while it is in place, and the need for multiple surgery events.[13] As a result, this technique is seldom used.

L5 Vertebrectomy

A more radical approach to gain reduction of the lumbar spine onto the sacrum is to perform an L5 vertebrectomy, fusing the L4 vertebra directly to the sacrum. This technique was developed by Gaines in 1979[14,15] because the contemporary techniques and instrumentation at the time were unable to adequately reduce the deformity. The surgical procedure is a 2-stage procedure:

Stage one:

- Anterior resection of L5 body and adjacent intervertebral discs

Stage two:

- Distraction to aid in the removal of the pedicles and posterior elements of L5
- Reduction of L4 onto the sacrum
- Compression applied from L4 to the sacrum via posterior instrumentation

Table 1
Details of high-grade dysplastic spondylolisthesis sagittal correction reported by prior studies, grouped by reduction technique used

Author, year	Reduction Technique	Preoperative Slip Angle	Postoperative Slip Angle	Preoperative LL	Postoperative LL	Preoperative PT	Postoperative PT	Preoperative SS/SI	Postoperative SS/SI	Preoperative CVA (cm)	Postoperative CVA (cm)	New Neurologic Deficits (%)	Pseudo (%)
Bradford & Boachie-Adjei,[11] 1990	Dome osteotomy, skeletal traction, then ALIF + cast	71	28	—	—	—	—	27	49	—	—	16	21
Smith et al,[32] 2001	Posterior distraction, partial reduction; transsacral screws	41	21	—	—	—	—	32	40	6.7	4.2	—	22
Shufflebarger & Geck,[19] 2005	SDO, posterior distraction, then instrument L5-S1 and compress	35	4	70	50	—	—	28	39	3.3	0.7	0	0
Ruf et al,[20] 2006	Posterior distraction, then instrument and compress	37	8	63	48	—	—	35	43	5.5	4.4	25	0
Karampalis et al,[13] 2012	External transpedicular fixation	67	23	—	—	43	19	17	27	—	—	22	11
Lehmer et al,[16] 1994	L5 vertebrectomy	48	−5	37	37	—	—	26	39	—	—	75	19

Min et al,[17] 2012	Sacral dome excision + TLIF	15	−6	69	42	25	28	51	48	—	—	27	0
Tian et al,[18] 2015	Sacral dome excision + reduction screws; TLIF	18	−7	35	50	38	28	33	44	—	—	8	0
Bouyer et al,[25] 2014	Transsacral rod fixation + cantilever	20	−12	70	52	37	30	38	47	—	—	42	0
Lamartina et al,[21] 2009	Schanz reduction screws	34	−2	"No change"	—	—	—	32	41	5.3	4.3	4	0
Martiniani et al,[22] 2012	Schanz reduction screws	—	—	—	—	41	30	36	47	—	—	20	0
Thomas et al,[23] 2015	Schanz reduction screws	20	−15	69	46	31	25	45	46	—	—	33	33
Average		36.9	3.3	—	—	—	—	—	—	—	—	23.3	8.8

Abbreviations: ALIF, anterior lumbar interbody fusion; CVA, cervical sagittal vertical axis; Pseudo, pseudarthrosis; SDO, sacral dome osteotomy; SI, sacral incidence.

Gaines[14] performed a follow-up study in 2005 evaluating 30 patients who underwent this procedure and noted that there was a high rate of solid arthrodesis; however, there was also an exceptionally high 77% incidence of L5 nerve deficits, although most of these ultimately recovered. Lehmer and colleagues[16] described the preoperative and postoperative sagittal parameters of 16 patients undergoing this procedure and found improvements in the sacral inclination (13°), although overall LL did not change. This study only had one patient with preoperative and postoperative films amenable to judge global alignment; however, in that one patient the T1 plumb line was brought from +46 mm to −3 mm over the posterior superior sacral endplate, evidencing a large correction.[16]

Sacral Dome Osteotomy

An osteotomy of the sacral dome is a technique that can be applied in conjunction with other techniques for improvement of the reduction. With HGDS, especially spondyloptosis, it is common to see abnormal rounded sacral endplate morphology, which is the result of chronic forces across the maloriented lumbosacral junction. This technique is typically performed from the posterior and creates flat sacral and inferior L5 endplates to facilitate reduction[17,18]:

- Wide decompression of L5-S1 with attention paid to the L5 nerve roots
- Anteriorly directed osteotomy of the S1 body is performed
- Additional osteotomy of the anterior inferior lip of the L5 body may be performed as needed

Min and colleagues[17] reported on a series of 15 patients undergoing this technique along with TLIF and posterior instrumentation (**Fig. 3**). In that series, it was noted that all of the patients preoperatively would meet Labelle type 4 classification (balanced pelvis), yet there was still an improvement in LL (decreased by 20°), although PT increased by 4°.[17] Tian and colleagues[18] also published results of 13 patients treated in a similar fashion and noted improvements in LL, SS, and PT. This technique is a useful adjunct in achieving a reduction and improving LL in patients with significant rounding/dysmorphism of the S1 endplate.

Posterior Distraction

Similar to an external fixation technique in which distraction is applied, intraoperative posterior distraction provides a focused application of force to the spondylolisthesis site, rather than relying on the global traction force provided by halo traction. An intuitive drawback to this technique would be the potential for iatrogenic hypolordosis, especially if fixation points for distraction are in the middle or cranial lumbar spine.

Shufflebarger and Geck[19] described a posterior distraction technique as follows (**Fig. 4**):

- Bilateral sacral alar hooks are connected to hooks in the middle to upper lumbar spine, which are used for temporary distraction to aid in exposure and reduction
- Sacral dome osteotomy performed
- Posterior lumbar interbody fusion (PLIF) of L5-S1 performed
- Pedicle screws are placed in L5 and the sacrum and compressed to provide a posterior lordosing force at that level
- Temporary distraction hooks are removed

In addition to facilitating reduction of the spondylolisthesis, this technique was efficacious in improving sagittal parameters, with Shufflebarger and Geck[19] reporting improvements in LL, SS, and sagittal vertical axis. Another study by Ruf and colleagues[20] also showed success in improving sagittal alignment with a similar technique, using temporary pedicle screws in L4 to provide distraction and reduction of L5.

Transpedicular L4/5 Reduction Screws

Modern instrumentation can be used to assist with intraoperative reductions. The following technique was used by Lamartina and colleagues[21]:

- Pedicle screws are placed into the S1 body
- Double-threaded Schanz pins are placed in transpedicular fashion into L5
- After locking 2 rods in place on the sacral screws, the Schanz pins are used to perform the reduction by utilization of the double thread, held against the immobile rod

Currently manufactured reduction pedicle screws can act in a similar fashion, allowing for posterior translation of L5 with respect to a rod fixed to sacral screws.[18] Several studies have evidenced the ability of this technique to achieve improvement in sagittal parameters of the spine.[21–23]

Ruf and colleagues[20] described temporary transpedicular instrumentation of L4 as a means to provide distraction from L4-S1 followed by reduction of L5 by pulling it dorsally with a reduction pedicle screw (**Fig. 5**). They noted excellent correction at follow-up with a reduction in slip angle from 36.6° to 7.6° and an improvement in

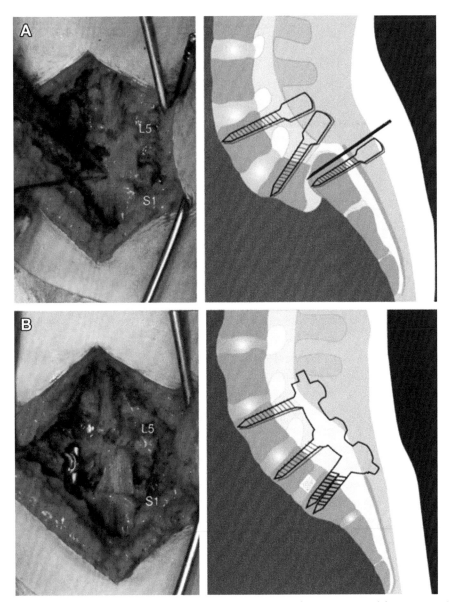

Fig. 3. (*A*) Sacral dome osteotomy from posterior using ordinary straight osteotomes. (*B*) Intraoperative photograph and drawing after the reduction. (*From* Min K, Liebscher T, Rothenfluh D. Sacral dome resection and single-stage posterior reduction in the treatment of high-grade high dysplastic spondylolisthesis in adolescents and young adults. Eur Spine J 2012;21(suppl 6):787; with permission.)

C7 plumb line from 55.4 mm to 44.1 mm at 2 years. There were 6 transient L5 nerve root deficits postoperatively, but no long-term motor deficits. However, they did have an almost 15% incidence of adjacent segment disease within 2 years, possibly related to extension of their dissection and instrumentation cranially.[20]

Cantilever Maneuver

A cantilever maneuver is commonly performed in cases of kyphosis throughout the spine.

Ilharreborde and colleagues[24] in 2007 applied to HGDS a method developed by Jackson for intra-sacral rod placement, allowing for a cantilever maneuver of the pelvis to the lumbar spine (**Fig. 6**) to create lordosis at the level of the spondylolisthesis:

- A sacral dome osteotomy is performed
- Pedicle screws are placed L4-S1
- Bilateral rods are then placed directly into the sacral alae caudal to the S1 pedicle screws, extending intraosseously to the level of S2 or

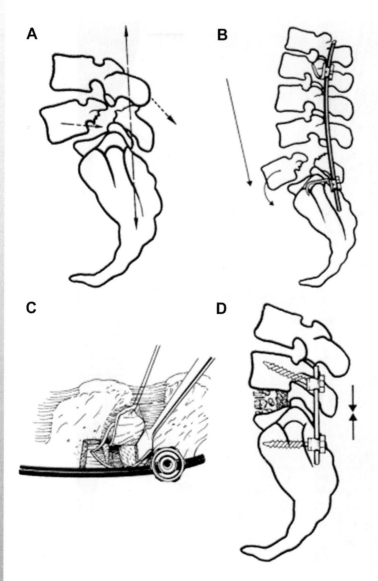

A

B

C

D

Fig. 4. The steps in reduction and PLIF. (*A*) A high dysplastic spondylolisthesis. (*B*) Temporary distraction using sacral alar hooks. Some improvement in sacral slip angle and in displacement is achieved. (*C*) Excision of the sacral dome, before placing the structural interbody graft. (*D*) Screw placement in the lumbar 5 and the sacrum, with rod placement, accomplishing reduction of the slip angle and of the percent displacement. Note the structural anterior interbody graft and the copious amount of autograft placed anterior to the Harm's cage. (*From* Shufflebarger HL, Geck MJ. High-grade isthmic dysplastic spondylolisthesis: monosegmental surgical treatment. Spine (Phila Pa 1976) 2005;30(6 suppl):S42–8; with permission.)

S3 to create an "iliac buttress" to resist distal cut-out during reduction

- With a cantilever maneuver, the sacrum can then be anteverted in the sagittal plane to reduce it to the L5 inferior endplate by locking the posterior rods into the L4 and L5 pedicle screw heads

A similar cantilever reduction can also be obtained with S2 alar-iliac pelvic screws, rather than burying the rods directly into the sacral ala. Bouyer and colleagues[25] reported consistent improvement in sagittal parameters with this maneuver. Notable from their series however was a higher rate of L5 nerve injury (42%), all of which ultimately recovered, and a high rate of wound complications (42%).[25]

Summary of Techniques

Of the multiple techniques that have been used for reduction, the 2 techniques that appear to most effectively correct the kyphosis of L5-S1 are external transpedicular fixation and L5 vertebrectomy, although both of these findings are reported in only one study, and a vertebrectomy carries an exceptionally high rate of neurologic injury. The remaining techniques are roughly similar in their ability to give lordosis to the L5-S1 level, each improving lordosis by 30° to 35°.

The techniques giving the highest overall change in LL are posterior distraction with temporary instrumentation, and the utilization of a cantilever reduction maneuver. Each modern technique has a similar effect on the

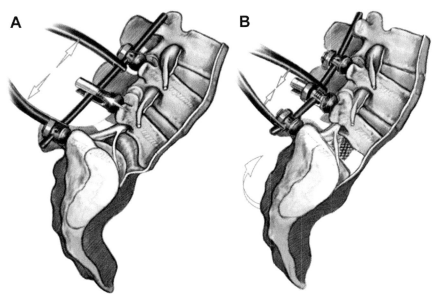

Fig. 5. Technique of reduction. (*A*) Reduction of slippage by distraction of L4-S1 and pulling back of L5. (*B*) Correction of kyphosis by posterior compression of L5-S1 against an anterior support. (*From* Ruf M, Koch H, Melcher RP, et al. Anatomic reduction and monosegmental fusion in high-grade developmental spondylolisthesis. Spine (Phila Pa 1976) 2006;31(3):269–74; with permission.)

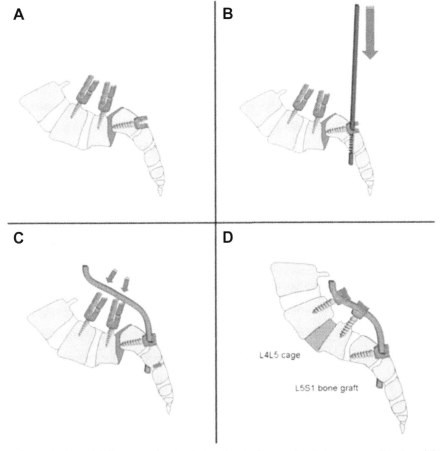

Fig. 6. Operative technique. (*A*) Intrasacral polyaxial and reduction, polyaxial screws positioning. (*B*) Transsacral rod positioning. (*C*) Progressive lumbosacral reduction using L4 and L5 reduction screws. (*D*) Final construct with L4-L5 posterior interbody fusion and L5-S1 anterior bone grafting by posterior approach. (*From* Bouyer B, Bachy M, Courvoisier A, et al. High-grade lumbosacral spondylolisthesis reduction and fusion in children using transsacral rod fixation. Child's Nerv Syst 2014;30(3):507; with permission.)

improvement of SS, although surprisingly the technique used by Bradford[11] in 1990 of a sacral dome osteotomy, 10 days of skeletal traction, followed by anterior interbody fusion gave more improvement in SS than any technique using modern instrumentation.

Authors' Preferred Surgical Technique

The authors' preferred technique (**Figs. 7** and **8**) uses several of the above techniques as part of a single-stage, posterior-only approach with circumferential arthrodesis via a TLIF, pelvic fixation, and a cantilever reduction maneuver:

- Patient positioned prone with their hips flexed in a leg sling
- Posted threaded reduction screws are placed through L5 pedicles
- Pedicle screws placed in S1, and L4 if necessary
  - Place S1 screws low in the pedicle to allow for sacral dome osteotomy
- Bilateral S2 alar-iliac screw placement
- Gill laminectomy at L5-S1
- L4 caudal hemilaminectomy performed to identify L5 nerve roots, which are followed out to the neuroforamina bilaterally
- L5-S1 diskectomy
- Sacral dome osteotomy
- L5-S1 transforaminal interbody fusion
  - Insert and rotate distractors used to elevate L5 for interbody cage placement
- Reduction
  - Rods locked to sacral screws
  - Hips are extended to antevert the pelvis, reducing the pelvis to the lumbar spine
  - Cantilever maneuver used to further reduce the pelvis to lumbar spine
    - This brings the rods into contact with the L4, L5 screw heads
  - Posted threaded reduction screws in the L5 body are used to persuade L5 posteriorly

- Assess reduction with intraoperative fluoroscopy
  - Primary goal is to restore lumbosacral lordosis
  - A full translational reduction is unnecessary
- Posterolateral spine fusion
  - Maximize decortication to achieve the greatest fusion surface area given the known hypoplastic transverse processes
- Postoperatively the patient is positioned on their side or supine with hips extended and knees bent to minimize L5 nerve root tension

The emphasis during this technique is on the restoration of lumbosacral lordosis, and a full translational reduction is not necessary. The authors wish to emphasize the concept of reducing the pelvis to the spine with a cantilever maneuver, rather than reducing the lumbar spine to the pelvis. In a situation whereby the L5 vertebra is reduced to a stationary pelvis, there is a potential for anterior pressure on the thecal sac, which could lead to a cauda equina syndrome. This risk is theoretically lowered by reducing the pelvis to a stationary lumbar spine.

COMPLICATIONS

The primary complications related to surgical management of HGDS are new neurologic deficits and pseudarthrosis.

New Neurologic Deficits

The most common injury is a postoperative deficit or radiculopathy of the L5 nerve root, unsurprising given the altered anatomy of the L5-S1 neural foramina and aberrant course of the L5 nerve roots in HGDS. Petraco and colleagues[26] illustrated that significant L5 nerve stretch occurs during reduction of HGDS, although notably the first half of reduction only produced 29% of the overall L5 nerve root strain. This concept makes a case to

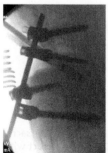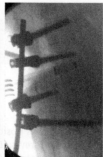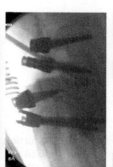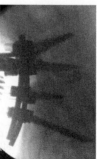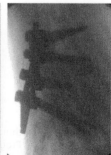

Fig. 7. Radiographic progression of reduction using the authors' preferred technique.

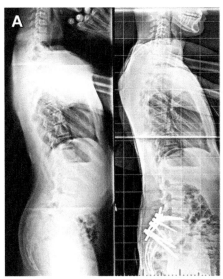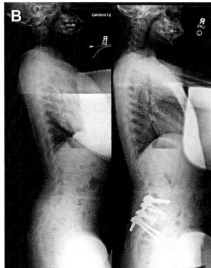

Fig. 8. Comparison of preoperative and postoperative radiographs following the authors' preferred technique on 2 (*A*, *B*) patients with spondyloptosis.

consider intentionally performing an incomplete reduction, as the L5 nerve root would see dramatically less strain than if a full reduction were performed.

A study of the Scoliosis Research Society database by Fu and colleagues[27] reviewed pediatric patients surgically treated for dysplastic spondylolisthesis. The findings from that study showed that there was a 10% rate of new neurologic deficit in the patients undergoing a reduction, compared with 2% in the patients who did not undergo reduction. However, a confounder to this finding is that more patients with preoperative neural compression symptoms underwent reduction, and subgroup analysis showed that those patients were at a much higher risk (10%) than those without a preoperative neural compressive symptom (1%). Thus, it is difficult to ascertain if the reduction or the presence of preoperative neurologic compressive symptoms is the true risk factor for a new postoperative neurologic deficit. Regarding the outcome of the new deficits, 50% attained a full recovery, 47% had a partial recovery, and 3% had no recovery.

A more recent review by Longo and colleagues[27] evaluated 8 studies on the surgical management of HGDS with either reduction or in situ fusion. The investigators found a similar rate of new neurologic deficit as Fu and colleagues[27] in patients undergoing reduction (7.8 vs 10%, respectively); however, the Longo study reported that the rate of neurologic deficit was not statistically different in patients treated with in situ fusion (7.8 vs 8.9% treated with in situ fusion).

Pseudarthrosis

Pseudarthrosis is a known complication in spondylolisthesis surgery, occurring in patients with in situ fusion and fusion after reduction.[8,28] Two systematic reviews both concluded that reduction results in a significantly lower rate of pseudarthrosis, with Longo reporting a rate of 5.5% in patients with a reduction compared with 17.8% of in situ fusions.[8,28]

Transvertebral transsacral strut grafting appears to improve the rate of solid arthrodesis for in situ fusions, although again this has been shown to not significantly change sagittal parameters.[29–31] Posterior instrumentation with a transsacral strut grafting technique can also be used after a partial reduction.[32]

SUMMARY

A modern understanding of the impact of HGDS on overall sagittal parameters helps to inform us as to which patients will benefit most from reduction at the time of fusion. Patients classified as Labelle types 5 or 6 merit strong consideration for reduction, as an in situ fusion will commit them to the unbalanced sagittal contour they rest in preoperatively. During reduction, the emphasis must be placed on restoration of lordosis, rather than focusing on translation. A cantilever reduction of the pelvis to the lumbar spine theoretically decreases the risk of a cauda equina syndrome. Reduction lowers the pseudarthrosis rate and does not significantly increase the rate of L5 nerve injury. Most reduction techniques are similar in their ability to impart lordosis to the L5-S1 level.

REFERENCES

1. Pawar A, Labelle H, Mac-Thiong J-M. The evaluation of lumbosacral dysplasia in young patients with lumbosacral spondylolisthesis: comparison with controls and relationship with the severity of slip. Eur Spine J 2012;21(11):2122–7.

2. Harris IE, Weinstein SL. Long-term follow-up of patients with grade-III and IV spondylolisthesis. Treatment with and without posterior fusion. J Bone Joint Surg Am 1987;69(7):960–9.

3. Labelle H, Roussouly P, Berthonnaud E, et al. Spondylolisthesis, pelvic incidence, and spinopelvic balance: a correlation study. Spine (Phila Pa 1976) 2004;29(18):2049–54.

4. Labelle H, Mac-Thiong J-M, Roussouly P. Spino-pelvic sagittal balance of spondylolisthesis: a review and classification. Eur Spine J 2011;20(Suppl 5):641–6.

5. Hresko MT, Labelle H, Roussouly P, et al. Classification of high-grade spondylolistheses based on pelvic version and spine balance: possible rationale for reduction. Spine (Phila Pa 1976) 2007;32(20):2208–13.

6. Harroud A, Labelle H, Joncas J, et al. Global sagittal alignment and health-related quality of life in lumbosacral spondylolisthesis. Eur Spine J 2013;22(4):849–56.

7. Blondel B, Schwab F, Ungar B, et al. Impact of magnitude and percentage of global sagittal plane correction on health-related quality of life at 2-years follow-up. Neurosurgery 2012;71(2):341–8.

8. Longo UG, Loppini M, Romeo G, et al. Evidence-based surgical management of spondylolisthesis: reduction or arthrodesis in situ. J Bone Joint Surg Am 2014;96(1):53–8.

9. Agabegi SS, Fischgrund JS. Contemporary management of isthmic spondylolisthesis: pediatric and adult. Spine J 2010;10(6):530–43.

10. Scaglietti O, Frontino G, Bartolozzi P. Technique of anatomical reduction of lumbar spondylolisthesis and its surgical stabilization. Clin Orthop Relat Res 1976;(117):165–75.

11. Bradford DS, Boachie-Adjei O. Treatment of severe spondylolisthesis by anterior and posterior reduction and stabilization. A long-term follow-up study. J Bone Joint Surg Am 1990;72(7):1060–6.

12. Magerl FP. Stabilization of the lower thoracic and lumbar spine with external skeletal fixation. Clin Orthop Relat Res 1984;(189):125–41.

13. Karampalis C, Grevitt M, Shafafy M, et al. High-grade spondylolisthesis: gradual reduction using Magerl's external fixator followed by circumferential fusion technique and long-term results. Eur Spine J 2012;21(Suppl 2):S200–6.

14. Gaines RW. L5 vertebrectomy for the surgical treatment of spondyloptosis: thirty cases in 25 years. Spine (Phila Pa 1976) 2005;30(6 Suppl):S66–70.

15. Gaines RW, Nichols WK. Treatment of spondyloptosis by two stage L5 vertebrectomy and reduction of L4 onto S1. Spine (Phila Pa 1976) 1985;10(7):680–6.

16. Lehmer SM, Steffee AD, Gaines RW Jr. Treatment of L5-S1 spondyloptosis by staged L5 resection with reduction and fusion of L4 onto S1 (Gaines procedure). Spine (Phila Pa 1976) 1994;19(17):1916–25.

17. Min K, Liebscher T, Rothenfluh D. Sacral dome resection and single-stage posterior reduction in the treatment of high-grade high dysplastic spondylolisthesis in adolescents and young adults. Eur Spine J 2012;21(Suppl 6):S785–91.

18. Tian W, Han X-G, Liu B, et al. Posterior reduction and monosegmental fusion with intraoperative three-dimensional navigation system in the treatment of high-grade developmental spondylolisthesis. Chin Med J (Engl) 2015;128(7):865–70.

19. Shufflebarger HL, Geck MJ. High-grade isthmic dysplastic spondylolisthesis: monosegmental surgical treatment. Spine (Phila Pa 1976) 2005;30(6 Suppl):S42–8.

20. Ruf M, Koch H, Melcher RP, et al. Anatomic reduction and monosegmental fusion in high-grade developmental spondylolisthesis. Spine (Phila Pa 1976) 2006;31(3):269–74.

21. Lamartina C, Zavatsky JM, Petruzzi M, et al. Novel concepts in the evaluation and treatment of high-dysplastic spondylolisthesis. Eur Spine J 2009;18(Suppl 1):133–42.

22. Martiniani M, Lamartina C, Specchia N. "In situ" fusion or reduction in high-grade high dysplastic developmental spondylolisthesis (HDSS). Eur Spine J 2012;21(Suppl 1):S134–40.

23. Thomas D, Bachy M, Courvoisier A, et al. Progressive restoration of spinal sagittal balance after surgical correction of lumbosacral spondylolisthesis before skeletal maturity. J Neurosurg Spine 2015;22(3):294–300.

24. Ilharreborde B, Fitoussi F, Morel E, et al. Jackson's intrasacral fixation in the management of high-grade isthmic spondylolisthesis. J Pediatr Orthop B 2007;16(1):16–8.

25. Bouyer B, Bachy M, Courvoisier A, et al. High-grade lumbosacral spondylolisthesis reduction and fusion in children using transsacral rod fixation. Childs Nerv Syst 2014;30(3):505–13.

26. Petraco DM, Spivak JM, Cappadona JG, et al. An anatomic evaluation of L5 nerve stretch in spondylolisthesis reduction. Spine (Phila Pa 1976) 1996;21(10):1133–8.

27. Fu K-MG, Smith JS, Polly DW, et al. Morbidity and mortality associated with spinal surgery in children: a review of the Scoliosis Research Society morbidity and mortality database: clinical article. J Neurosurg Pediatr 2011;7(1):37–41.

28. Transfeldt EE, Mehbod AA. Evidence-based medicine analysis of isthmic spondylolisthesis treatment

including reduction versus fusion in situ for high-grade slips. Spine (Phila Pa 1976) 2007;32(19 Suppl):S126–9.

29. Bohlman HH, Cook SS. One-stage decompression and posterolateral and interbody fusion for lumbosacral spondyloptosis through a posterior approach. Report of two cases. J Bone Joint Surg Am 1982; 64(3):415–8.

30. Sasso RC, Shively KD, Reilly TM. Transvertebral transsacral strut grafting for high-grade isthmic spondylolisthesis L5-S1 with fibular allograft. J Spinal Disord Tech 2008;21(5):328–33.

31. Lengert R, Charles YP, Walter A, et al. Posterior surgery in high-grade spondylolisthesis. Orthop Traumatol Surg Res 2014;100(5):481–4.

32. Smith JA, Deviren V, Berven S, et al. Clinical outcome of trans-sacral interbody fusion after partial reduction for high-grade L5-S1 spondylolisthesis. Spine (Phila Pa 1976) 2001;26(20): 2227–34.

Sacropelvic Fixation
When, Why, How?

Joseph M. Lombardi, MD*, Jamal N. Shillingford, MD, Lawrence G. Lenke, MD,
Ronald A. Lehman, MD

KEYWORDS

• Sacropelvic • Pelvic • Fixation • S2AI • Deformity

KEY POINTS

- The indications for sacropelvic fixation continue to evolve with emerging instrumentation technologies and advancing techniques.
- Common indications include long construct fusions, high-grade spondylolisthesis, sacral fractures, sacral tumors, and global sagittal and/or coronal imbalance among others.
- The authors' preferred technique is through use of a freehand S2-alar-iliac screw placement.

INTRODUCTION

Continued advancements in surgical techniques and instrumentation technology have allowed surgeons to make great strides in the treatment of adult spinal deformity. Many challenges remain, including lumbosacral pseudoarthrosis and fixation failure, with no clear consensus on the best indications or techniques for sacropelvic fixation. Nonetheless, there is a continued movement toward the utilization of robust sacropelvic fixation as a necessary tool for sagittal and coronal correction in advanced deformity. This article seeks to provide background on the historical development, biomechanics, and modern techniques associated with the use of sacropelvic fixation in treating adult spinal deformity.

ANATOMIC AND BIOMECHANICAL CONSIDERATIONS

An understanding of lumbosacral anatomy and biomechanics is paramount when considering appropriate construct selection for instrumentation to the pelvis. It also helps to explain the shortcomings of historical fixation techniques. The lumbosacral junction is subject to shear forces as high as 100 N during bending, which must be accounted for when attempting fusion across this segment.[1] McCord and colleagues[2] first introduced the concept of a biomechanical lumbosacral pivot point. This was defined as the central axis at the middle osteoligamentous column between the last lumbar vertebra and the sacrum (**Fig. 1**). The study demonstrated the importance in the relationship between the sacropelvic fixation points and the lumbosacral pivot, where construct stability increases as fixation progresses ventral to the pivot point. O'Brien[3] postulated that sacral fixation can be defined in terms of 3 anatomic zones (**Fig. 2**). Zone 1 is defined as the S1 vertebral body, including the cephalad sacral alae. Zone 2 spans from the caudad sacral alae, through the S2 vertebral body down to the tip of the coccyx. Last, zone 3 represents the ilia. These zones carry clinical significance in that construct stability improves as fixation moves caudally through the zones with zone 3 affording the greatest biomechanical resistance to pull out. Likewise, instrumentation through the ilium allows for fixation points anterior to the lumbosacral pivot point further enhancing stability.

Disclosure: The authors have nothing to disclose.
Department of Orthopaedic Surgery, Columbia University Medical Center, The Spine Hospital at New York Presbyterian, 5141 Broadway, 3 Field West, New York, NY 10034, USA
* Corresponding author.
E-mail address: jml2285@cumc.columbia.edu

Neurosurg Clin N Am 29 (2018) 389–397
https://doi.org/10.1016/j.nec.2018.02.001

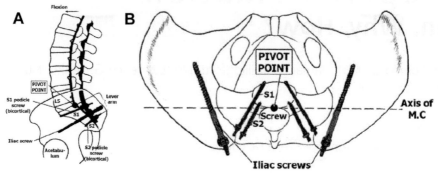

Fig. 1. (*A*) The lumbosacral pivot point seen on sagittal view. (*B*) Axial illustration of the lumbosacral pivot point. M.C, Middle osteoligamentous column. (*From* Moshirfar A, Rand FF, Sponseller PD, et al. Pelvic fixation in spine surgery. Historical overview, indications, biomechanical relevance, and current techniques. J Bone Joint Surg Am 2005;87(Suppl 2):89–106; with permission.)

HISTORICAL PERSPECTIVE
Early Twentieth Century

The first known description of posterior spinal instrumentation dates to 1891 when B.A. Hadra published a technique article describing the wiring of multiple cervical spinous processes to serve as a "resistant posterior brace" following a fracture-dislocation in a patient with Pott disease.[4] In 1910, Fritz Lange described the use of steel rods as a means of stabilizing a spondylotic spine.[5] Russel Hibbs of the New York Orthopaedic Hospital and Fred Albee worked independently to describe the first reports of spinal arthrodesis for the treatment of Pott disease, which they concurrently published in 1911.[6,7] The Hibbs technique of local autograft to achieve fusion served as a fundamental building block for spinal fusion advancements for decades to come. Despite its implementation in extrapulmonary tuberculosis,

Hibbs postulated that this technique could be used for scoliosis as well. He later published on this in 1924, when he described the use of spinal fusion for the treatment of scoliosis in 45 patients.[8] Of note, 3 of those patients had lumbosacral fusions performed. Interestingly, Hibbs[9] identified the lumbosacral junction as the "point of greatest strain" in the normal spine and advocated for lumbosacral fusion in specific instances. Variations of the Hibbs technique were described in years to come, notably among them by Alexander Forbes, who described denuding the spinous process and lamina in order to achieve in situ fusion. In 1933, Ralph Ghormley described lumbosacral fusion for the treatment of symptomatic lumbosacral spondylosis.[10] He believed that the high sheer forces between the lumbar spine and fixed sacrum accounted for most lower back pain. In addition, Ghormley[11] was the first to describe the use of iliac

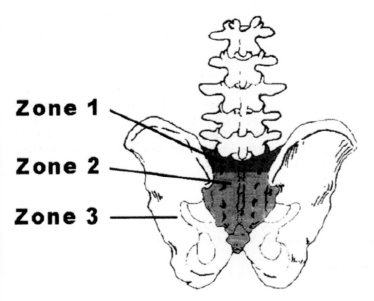

Fig. 2. Zones of sacropelvic fixation. (*From* Arlet V, Carl AL, O'Brien MF, et al. Sacropelvic fixation in spinal deformity. In: DeWald RL, editor. Spinal deformities: the comprehensive text. New York: Thieme; 2003. p. 601–14; with permission.)

crest bone graft as an adjuvant for lumbosacral fusion, a technique that remains in use to this day. However, it was not until the 1940s when King[12] and Toumey[13] were the first to perform concurrent instrumentation with autologous bone grafting for fusion. King's technique entailed the use of transarticular screws across the facets in order to provide rigid fixation in an attempt to obviate postoperative bracing.

Advent of Rigid Instrumentation

Despite steady advancements in both fusion technique and spinal instrumentation in the early twentieth century, the mainstay of achieving lumbosacral fusion before the 1960s was through in situ bone grafting and prolonged cast immobilization. However, outcomes using this immobilization technique were poor, with pseudarthrosis rates approaching 50% in some studies.[13] Paul Harrington developed the first system for rigid spinal fixation for the treatment of scoliosis, which was introduced in the early 1960s.[14] This system relied on hooks at the cephalad and caudal transverse processes or laminae, which would effect distraction on the spinal column. Despite its early acceptance, this system did have significant shortcomings because of the fact that fixation was uniplanar and dependent on distraction. This was especially marked across the lumbosacral junction, where pseudarthrosis rates were reported to be as high as 40%.[15,16] Other complications of this construct included high rates of sacral hook dislodgement and loss of lumbar lordosis resulting in "flat back" syndrome.[17]

Eduardo Luque sought to address failures of Harrington hook and rod system by introducing instrumentation that used multiple points of rigid fixation throughout the construct.[18] This was accomplished by use of sublaminar wires, which were affixed to a 6.4-mm rod providing segmental fixation. Luque and Cardoso[19] introduced a curve into the cephalad and caudal aspect of the rods known as the "L rod" in an attempt to prevent migration. Advantages of this system included correction in both coronal and sagittal planes, unlike the prior Harrington fixation method. However, despite multiple points of fixation, rigidity across the lumbosacral junction, which is subject to large bending forces, proved to be inadequate in many circumstances with pseudarthrosis rates ranging from 6% to 41%.[20,21]

The 1980s offered further advancements in rigid spinal fixation with the development of the Cotrel-Dubousset (CD) instrumentation system.[22] This CD instrumentation system made use of monoaxial pedicle screws as well as hooks in order to provide multiple points of fixation to the distal spine. The increased rigidity of this construct allowed for the introduction of axial derotation, permitting 3-dimensional correction in patients with advanced idiopathic and de novo scoliosis.[23] Despite the technical advancement of the CD system, lumbosacral fixation with monoaxial pedicle screws at the sacrum offered inadequate fixation relative to the significant biomechanical shear forces across the lumbosacral junction.[23] This resulted in published rates of lumbosacral pseudarthrosis as high as 33% with pullout of sacral pedicle screws approaching 44%.[24] Allen and Ferguson,[25,26] who first described the Galveston Iliac Rod technique in 1983, sought to achieve rigid fixation across the lumbosacral junction by inserting L-shaped rods into the ilium from the posterior superior iliac spine (PSIS). The rod was tunneled submuscularly and achieved pelvic fixation between the inner and outer tables of the ilium. This construct resulted in improved pseudarthrosis rates relative to sacral pedicle screw fixation alone.[27,28] However, because of the superficial starting point in the PSIS, the Galveston technique presented challenges with implant prominence. In addition, loosening of the rods secondary to micromotion has been reported resulting in pain and the characteristic "windshield wiper" effect, which can be seen radiographically.[29]

MODERN TECHNIQUES

Iliac screw fixation represents a common technique for lumbopelvic fixation used by many surgeons in practice today. It offers distinct advantages over the traditional Galveston rod method, namely, through higher pullout strength and a greater degree of freedom in choosing the insertion point. Iliac screws can be inserted anywhere along the ilium, independent of other points of fixation and subsequently attached to a long construct through connectors. This modularity allows for the placement of multiple iliac screws on each side of the construct. In addition, Schwend and colleagues[30] demonstrated a 3-fold increase in pullout strength when compared with Galveston rods. This is likely attributed to the fact that iliac screw fixation is established in a divergent coronal plane relative to the rest of the construct, allowing for greater resistance to distal pullout. However, iliac screws pose a unique set of challenges as demonstrated by Tsuchiya and colleagues,[31] who described 34% of patients requiring removal of iliac screws following fusion for adult spinal deformity. In addition, insertion of the screws places the contents of the sciatic notch, including the superior gluteal artery and sciatic nerve at risk.

Last, iliac screws may also require extensive soft tissue dissection, which increases the risk of infection upwards of 4% as demonstrated by Kulko and colleagues.[32]

The use of sacral pedicle screws as the primary means of lumbosacral fixation is not recommended because of rates of failure as high as 44%.[24] This is likely attributed to the wide diameter of the sacral pedicles and lack of cancellous bone. In addition, the inclusion of S2 pedicle screws does not offer increased pullout strength when added to an S1 construct. This is likely due to the fact that the S2 pedicle is dorsal to the sacral pivot point.[2] Lehman and colleagues[33] demonstrated that sacral pedicle screw pullout strength can be improved through tricortical fixation, which can be achieved by directing the screw trajectory into the cortical bone of the sacral promontory. Likewise, screws directed 45° laterally into the sacral ala offer increased pullout strength versus standard sacral pedicle screws.[34] The application of sacral promontory and sacral alar screws does require a degree of technical expertise because the safe zones for insertion are narrow.[35] Despite the biomechanical advantages of such sacral fixation techniques, the use of sacral screws in isolation has poor clinical results and high rates of pseudarthrosis when used in long fusion constructs.[34]

S2-alar-iliac (S2AI) screw fixation for sacropelvic fixation was first described by Sponseller[36] and Kebaish[37] in 2007 for use in pediatric and adult spinal deformity and has increased in popularity since that time. S2AI screws offer many advantages to prior techniques in that they provide stable pelvic fixation that is in line with S1 screws and less prominent, without the additional dissection required for traditional iliac screws. Chang and colleagues[38] demonstrated a starting point for the S2AI screw that is 15 mm deeper than an entry point for the PSIS, reducing implant prominence for this fixation method. The classic description of S2AI screw insertion is through a start point that is between the S1 and S2 foramen with the screw trajectory aimed laterally 40° in the axial plane and 20° to 25° caudally in the sagittal plane.[39,40] However, these values have been shown to vary based on pelvic tilt and transitional sacral anatomy.[40] This technique takes advantage of the visible and palpable anatomic landmarks around the sacrum and pelvis, which allows for accurate and reproducible screw insertion.[41] The fact that the screw is placed in line with the S1 screw obviates rod connectors and allows for easier rod insertion. The S2AI method has also recently been described through a percutaneous approach by Martin and colleagues.[42] In addition,

Laratta and colleagues[43] demonstrated the safety and feasibility of robotic-assisted S2AI screw placement.

In an attempt to further reduce the risk of pseudarthrosis and rod breakage, various authors have described the use of multiple rod techniques or the placement of 3 to 4 iliac screws. The use of a "4-rod" technique as described by Shen and colleagues[44] has been proven to be biomechanically superior to traditional 2-rod constructs. However, this technique is technically challenging because it requires pedicle screw placement at different angles throughout the construct. It is the practice of the senior authors to routinely use additional rods in long fusion constructs particularly when poor bone quality and potential for fusion are of concern. In addition, the authors have begun to use ancillary rods to assist in instances of severe coronal imbalance, which cannot be addressed through traditional corrective techniques. This "kickstand" rod requires distal fixation at the ilium through traditional iliac screw insertion at the iliac crest. A rod is then connected to the proximal aspect of the curve through connectors and distracted across its length in order to establish a balanced hemipelvis (**Fig. 3**).

INDICATIONS FOR SACROPELVIC FIXATION

The indications for sacropelvic fixation continue to evolve as improving surgical techniques and implant technologies emerge. However, there are clinical instances in which sacropelvic fixation provides clear advantages in the pursuit of achieving construct stability and bony union. Conditions in which sacropelvic fixation is commonly used include high-grade spondylolisthesis, long fusion constructs, sacral fractures, sacral tumors, flat back deformities, 3-column osteotomies, and correction of pelvic obliquity.

There is no clear consensus in the literature as to the definition of a long fusion construct. Classic teaching defines long fusions as any construct that extends cephalad to the L2 vertebral body.[45–48] However, more conservative definitions include instrumentation that extends to the thoracolumbar spine.[45–48] Nonetheless, it is a prudent practice for the surgeon to consider sacropelvic fixation anytime instrumentation is extended into the sacrum. Likewise, an intraoperative clinical assessment should be made with respect to the integrity of sacral fixation, bone quality, and presence of sacral fractures when determining the need for further pelvic instrumentation. Coronal and sagittal balance should additionally be taken into consideration as to not place excessive stress along the L5-S1 segment leading to rapid degeneration. Such

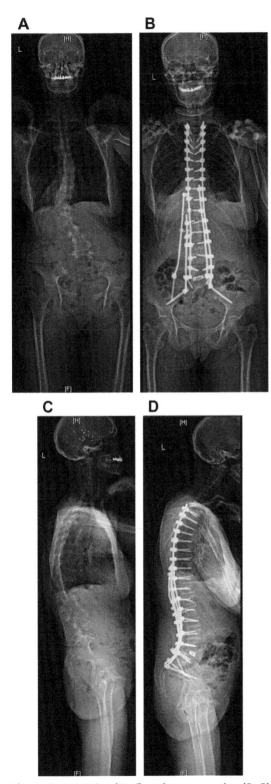

conditions include adult de novo scoliosis, idiopathic scoliosis with structural thoracolumbar or lumbar curves (**Fig. 4**), fixed kyphoscoliosis with significant sagittal imbalance (**Fig. 5**), flat back deformity from prior Harrington instrumentation, and neuromuscular scoliosis. Last, one should consider sacropelvic fixation whenever performing lumbar 3-column osteotomies.

High-grade spondylolisthesis (grade 3 or higher) at the caudal lumbar spine requires instrumentation to the sacrum to achieve reduction and fixation of the unstable segment. However,

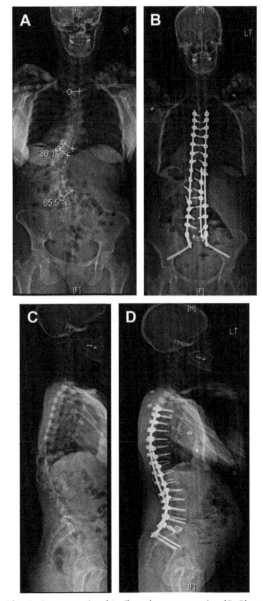

Fig. 3. Preoperative (*A*, *C*) and postoperative (*B*, *D*) films demonstrate use of a "kickstand" construct in a patient with progressive thoracolumbar and lumbosacral degenerative scoliosis with a 4-cm left-sided coronal imbalance.

Fig. 4. Preoperative (*A*, *C*) and postoperative (*B*, *D*) radiographs of sacropelvic fixation for adult idiopathic scoliosis with a structural lumbar curve.

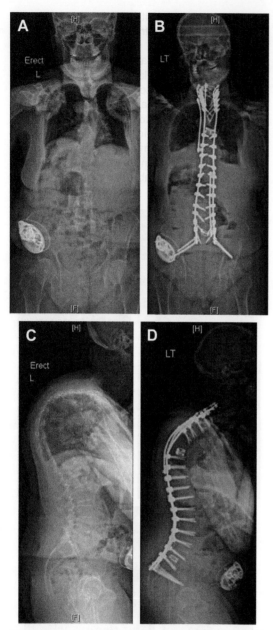

Fig. 5. Preoperative (*A, C*) and postoperative (*B, D*) films demonstrating 3 column osteotomies and sacropelvic fixation for the treatment of severe, fixed kyphoscoliosis resulting in thoracic myelopathy.

biomechanical studies have demonstrated large pullout forces placed on distal sacral fixation for the treatment of this condition.[49] Because of this, sacropelvic fixation is often advocated for in an attempt to reduce screw failure and undue rates of pseudarthrosis.

Less common indications for sacropelvic instrumentation include sacral fragility fractures in osteoporotic patients, sacral fractures secondary to high-energy trauma, and stabilization after excision

of sacral tumors.[50,51] Last, correction of pelvic obliquity as seen most commonly in patients with neuromuscular scoliosis can be an indication for sacropelvic fixation.

AUTHORS' PREFERRED TECHNIQUE

The use of S2AI screws has been adopted as the preferred method of sacropelvic fixation at the authors' institution. Although varying techniques for S2AI screw placement have been described in the literature, that is, fluoroscopic and robotic assisted, it is the authors' belief that when used correctly, a freehand S2AI technique is easily reproducible, efficient, and safe. The S2AI screw is most easily inserted from the contralateral side of the patient. The initial step to free hand screw placement begins with meticulous subperiosteal dissection of the posterior elements of the cephalad sacrum to expose anatomic landmarks, including the S2AI starting point, while also palpating the most distal portion of the PSIS with the bovie tip. The entry point is located just lateral to the midpoint of the S1 and S2 foramen and should be in line with the S1 screw (**Fig. 6**). A 3.5-mm acorn-tipped burr is used to establish a 5-mm-deep cortical breach at the screw entry point. A 2-mm blunt-tipped pedicle probe is advanced toward the sacroiliac (SI) joint with the curved tip directed posteriorly to avoid anterior perforation. The pedicle probe is directed toward the anterior inferior iliac spine (AIIS) by aiming to a point just cephalad to the posterior distal edge of the PSIS and perpendicular to the lateral sacral crest, which avoids the sciatic notch inferiorly. When the pedicle probe passes the hard cortical surface of the SI joint, at a depth of about 50 mm, it is removed and the bony channel is palpated with a flexible ball-tipped pedicle sounding or palpating instrument to assess for pelvic wall perforation. Ball-tip probing should confirm an intraosseous trajectory for the screw with the presence of a floor and 4 intact bony walls (anterior, posterior, superior, and inferior). The pedicle probe is then reinserted at the original depth, rotated to face anteriorly, and carefully placed into the base of the hole. The probe should be advanced toward the AIIS in a smooth and consistent manner to a depth of about 70 to 90 mm with a trajectory that keeps the tip of the probe heading in a more anterior position. Another helpful anatomic trajectory tip is to aim the probe just cephalad to the distal PSIS to avoid hitting the sciatic notch. Any sudden advancement or concern for cortical breach can be assessed with ball-tip probing of the bony floor and walls. The ball-tip probe is also used to document screw length with a

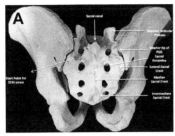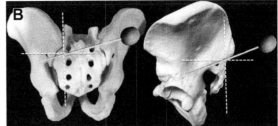

Fig. 6. (*A*) Posterior sacropelvic anatomy. (*B*) Pedicle probe trajectory in the coronal and sagittal plane. (*From* Shillingford JN, Laratta JL, Tan LA, et al. The free-hand technique for S2-alar-iliac screw placement: a safe and effective method for sacropelvic fixation in adult spinal deformity. J Bone Joint Surg Am 2018;100(4):334–342; with permission.)

hemostat clamp. If cortical perforation into soft tissue is noted, the screw path can be salvaged by redirecting the pedicle probe in a more appropriate direction, typically in a more medial and/or caudad position. The S2AI trajectory is undertapped 1 to 2 mm less than the desired screw diameter only if more than one screw pathway had been created (usually 8.5 × 90-mm screws are used). Tapping is performed with a cannulated tap over a K-wire, ensuring first that a bony floor is present to avoid damage to any soft tissue or neurovascular structures distal to the screw path. The intraosseous path and screw length are confirmed once more using the ball-tip probe and a hemostat to compare length directly to the chosen screw. The screw is then inserted (typically with a powered drill) in the direction of the established S2AI path. The optimal position of the screw lies immediately superior to the sciatic notch within the thick cortical bone of the ilium, which provides increased pullout strength along with the cortical bone of the sacrum and ilium as the screw traverses the SI joint.

In cases where 2 screws are desired on a single side of the hemipelvis, the space between the S1 and S2 foramen is divided in half before screw insertion. The first screw insertion site is centered at the top half near the S1 foramen using the previously described technique, whereas the second screw insertion site is centered at the bottom half near the S2 foramen.

SUMMARY

The indications for sacropelvic fusion continue to evolve as advancements in surgical technique and technologies continue to emerge in the literature. However, common indications for sacropelvic fixation include long construct fusions, high-grade spondylolisthesis, sacral fractures, sacral tumors, and global sagittal and/or coronal imbalance, among others. Currently, multiple feasible techniques for sacropelvic fixation exist

in the literature; however, it is the preferred technique of the authors' to perform S2AI fixation by means of freehand technique, which has proven safe and effective.

REFERENCES

1. Kornblatt MD, Casey MP, Jacobs RR. Internal fixation in lumbosacral spine fusion. Clin Orthop Relat Res 1986;(203):141–50.
2. McCord DH, Cunningham BW, Shono Y, et al. Biomechanical analysis of lumbosacral fixation. Spine (Phila Pa 1976) 1992;17(8 Suppl):S235–43.
3. O'Brien MF. Sacropelvic fixation in spinal deformity. In: DeWald RL, editor. Spinal deformities: the comprehensive text. New York: Thieme; 2003. p. 601–14.
4. Hadra BE. Wiring the spinous processes in Pott's disease. Trans Am Orthopassoc 1891;4:206–10.
5. Lange F, Peltier LF. The classic. Support for the spondylitic spine by means of 6. buried steel bars, attached to the vertebrae. By Fritz Lange. 1910. Clin Orthop Relat Res 1986;(203):3–6.
6. Hibbs RA. An operation for progressive spinal deformities: a preliminary report of three cases from the service of the orthopaedic hospital. New York Med J 1911;93(21):1013–6.
7. Albee FH. Transplantation of a portion of the tibia into the spine for Pott's disease. A preliminary report. J Am Med Assoc 1911;57:885–6.
8. Hibbs RA. A report of fifty-nine cases of scoliosis treated by the fusion operation. By Russell A. Hibbs, 1924. Clin Orthop Relat Res 1988;(229):4–19.
9. Mackenzie Forbes A. Technique of an operation for spinal fusion as practised in Montreal. J Orthop Surg 1920;2(9):509–14.
10. Ghormley RK. Low back pain with special reference to the articular facets, with presentation of an operative procedure. JAMA 1933;101(23):1773–7.
11. King D. Internal fixation for lumbosacral fusion. J Bone Joint Surg Am 1948;30:560–5.
12. Toumey JW. The simplification of spine fusion technic by use of the bone bank. Lahey Clin Bull 1949;6:162–6.

13. Thompson WA, Ralston EL. Pseudoarthrosis following spine fusion. J Bone Joint Surg Am 1949;31:400–5.

14. Harrington PR. Treatment of scoliosis. Correction and internal fixation by spine instrumentation. J Bone Joint Surg Am 1962;44:591–610.

15. Kostuik JP. Treatment of scoliosis in the adult thoracolumbar spine with special reference to fusion to the sacrum. Orthop Clin North Am 1988;19:371–81.

16. Devlin VJ, Asher MA. Biomechanics and surgical principles of long fusions to the sacrum. Spine State Art Rev 1996;10:515–44.

17. Balderston RA, Winter RB, Moe JH, et al. Fusion to the sacrum for nonparalytic scoliosis in the adult. Spine 1986;11:824–9.

18. Luque ER, Cardoso A. Segmental correction of scoliosis with rigid internal fixation, a preliminary report. Orthop Trans 1977;1:136–7.

19. Luque ER. Segmental spinal instrumentation for correction of scoliosis. Clin Orthop Relat Res 1982;(163):192–8.

20. Boachie-Adjei O, Lonstein JE, Winter RB, et al. Management of neuromuscular spinal deformities with Luque segmental instrumentation. J Bone Joint Surg Am 1989;71(4):548–62.

21. Kostuik JP, Errico TJ, Gleason TF. Techniques of internal fixation for degenerative conditions of the lumbar spine. Clin Orthop Relat Res 1986;(203):219–31.

22. Cotrel Y, Dubousset J. New segmental posterior instrumentation of the spine. Orthop Trans 1985;9:118.

23. Camp JF, Caudle R, Ashmun RD, et al. Immediate complications of Cotrel-Dubousset instrumentation to the sacro-pelvis. A clinical and biomechanical study. Spine 1990;15:932–41.

24. Devlin VJ, Boachie-Adjei O, Bradford DS, et al. Treatment of adult spinal deformity with fusion to the sacrum using CD instrumentation. J Spinal Disord 1991;4:1–14.

25. Allen BL Jr, Ferguson RL. A pictorial guide to the Galveston LRI pelvic fixation technique. Contemp Orthop 1983;7(3):51–61.

26. Allen BL Jr, Ferguson RL. The Galveston experience with L-rod instrumentation for adolescent idiopathic scoliosis. Clin Orthop Relat Res 1988;(229):59–69.

27. Allen BL Jr, Ferguson RL. L rod instrumentation for scoliosis in cerebral palsy. J Pediatr Orthop 1982;2:87–96.

28. Saer EH III, Winter RB, Lonstein JE. Long scoliosis fusion to the sacrum in adults with nonparalytic scoliosis. An improved method. Spine (Phila Pa 1976) 1990;15:650–3.

29. Broom MJ, Banta JV, Renshaw TS. Spinal fusion augmented by Luque-rod segmental instrumentation for neuromuscular scoliosis. J Bone Joint Surg Am 1989;71:32–44.

30. Schwend RM, Sluyters R, Najdzionek J. The pylon concept of pelvic anchorage for spinal instrumentation in the human cadaver. Spine (Phila Pa 1976) 2003;28:542–7.

31. Tsuchiya K, Bridwell KH, Kuklo TR, et al. Minimum 5-year analysis of L5-S1 fusion using sacropelvic fixation (bilateral S1 and iliac screws) for spinal deformity. Spine (Phila Pa 1976) 2006;31(3):303–8.

32. Kuklo TR, Bridwell KH, Lewis SJ, et al. Minimum 2-year analysis of sacropelvic fixation and L5–S1 fusion using S1 and iliac screws. Spine (Phila Pa 1976) 2001;26:1976–83.

33. Lehman RA Jr, Kuklo TR, Belmont PJ Jr, et al. Advantage of pedicle screw fixation directed into the apex of the sacral promontory over bicortical fixation: a biomechanical analysis. Spine 2002;27:806–11.

34. Zindrick MR, Wiltse LL, Widell EH, et al. A biomechanical study of intrapeduncular screw fixation in the lumbosacral spine. Clin Orthop Relat Res 1986;(203):99–112.

35. Mirkovic S, Abitbol JJ, Steinman J, et al. Anatomic consideration for sacral screw placement. Spine (Phila Pa 1976) 1991;16:S289–94.

36. Sponseller PD. The S2 portal to the ilium. Roundtables Spine Surg 2007;2(2):83–7.

37. Kebaish KM. Sacropelvic fixation: techniques and complications. Spine (Phila Pa 1976) 2010;35(25):2245–51.

38. Chang TL, Sponseller PD, Kebaish KM, et al. Low profile pelvic fixation. Anatomic parameters for sacral alar-iliac fixation versus traditional iliac fixation. Spine (Phila Pa 1976) 2009;34:436–40.

39. Kebaish KM, Dafrawy M. Sacropelvic fixation. In: Vaccaro AR, Baron E, editors. Operative techniques: spine surgery. Philadelpia: Elsevier; 2016. p. 240–54.

40. Zhu F, Bao HD, Yuan S, et al. Posterior second sacral alar iliac screw insertion: anatomic study in a Chinese population. Eur Spine J 2013;22(7):1683–9.

41. Shillingford JN, Laratta JL, Tan LA, et al. The freehand technique for S2-alar-iliac screw placement:a safe and effective method for sacropelvic fixation in adult spinal deformity. J Bone Joint Surg Am 2018;100(4):334–42.

42. Martin CT, Witham TF, Kebaish KM. Sacropelvic fixation: two case reports of a new percutaneous technique. Spine (Phila Pa 1976) 2011;36(9):E618–21.

43. Laratta JL, Shillingford JN, Lombardi JM, et al. Accuracy of S2 alar-iliac screw placement under robotic guidance. Spine Deform 2018;6(2):130–6.

44. Shen FH, Harper M, Foster WC, et al. A novel "four-rod technique" for lumbo-pelvic reconstruction: theory and technical considerations. Spine 2006;31(12):1395–401.

45. Bridwell KH, Kuklo T, Edwards CC 2nd, et al. Sacropelvic fixation. Memphis (TN): Medtronic Sofamor Danek USA; 2004.

46. Perra JH. Techniques of instrumentation in long fusions to the sacrum. Orthop Clin North Am 1994;25:287–99.

47. Rosner MK, Ondra SL. Sacropelvic fixation in adult deformity. Sem Spine Surg 2004;16: 107–13.

48. Cunningham BW, Lewis SJ, Long J, et al. Biomechanical evaluation of lumbosacral reconstruction techniques for spondylolisthesis: an in vitro porcine model. Spine 2002;27:2321–7.

49. O'Brien MF, Kuklo TR, Mardjetko SJ, et al. The sacropelvic unit: creative solutions to complex fixation and reconstruction problems. Sem Spine Surg 2004;16:134–49.

50. Lourie H. Spontaneous osteoporotic fracture of the sacrum. An unrecognized syndrome of the elderly. JAMA 1982;248:715–7.

51. Gau YL, Lonstein JE, Winter RB, et al. Luque-Galveston procedure for correction and stabilization of neuromuscular scoliosis and pelvic obliquity: a review of 68 patients. J Spinal Disord 1991;4:399–410.

Evolution of the Minimally Invasive Spinal Deformity Surgery Algorithm
An Evidence-Based Approach to Surgical Strategies for Deformity Correction

Winward Choy, MD[a], Catherine A. Miller, MD[a],
Andrew K. Chan, MD[a], Kai-Ming Fu, MD[b],
Paul Park, MD[c], Praveen V. Mummaneni, MD[a],*

KEYWORDS

- MISDEF • Adult spinal deformity • Minimally invasive surgery • Scoliosis

KEY POINTS

- Minimally invasive deformity correction offers the potential to decrease surgical complications associated with open corrections.
- The MISDEF algorithm was developed to help identify appropriate candidates for MIS deformity correction using radiographic parameters.
- Additional factors such as clinical symptoms, pathology, and medical comorbidities must also be included in decision making for deformity patients.

INTRODUCTION

Adult spinal deformity (ASD) is a health care priority because the pathology is increasing in incidence with an aging US population, and affected patients have significant compromise in health status including pain and disability.[1–4] Thoracolumbar scoliosis and kyphosis are resultant from several pathologies including degenerative disk disease, rheumatoid arthritis, pre-existing deformity, trauma, infection, and iatrogenic causes.[5] Primary presenting symptoms include chronic back pain, deformity, and neurogenic claudication resultant from stenosis.[6] Although traditional open surgical techniques are effective in the treatment of ASD,[7,8] they are associated with a high rate of complications. Minimally invasive surgery (MIS) approaches to spinal deformity offer the potential to decrease surgical complications associated with open corrections.[9–11] MIS approaches are increasingly recognized as effective and save, with the opportunity to reduce trauma to soft tissue, decrease intraoperative blood loss, and minimize surgical site infections.[12–14] These advantages may be particularly critical in an

Disclosure Statement: Choy, Miller, Chan: no disclosures Park: royalties from Globus; consultant for Globus, NuVasive, Zimmer Biomet, and Medtronic. Fu: consultant for SI-BONE. Devin: consultant for Stryker Spine and Medtronic; clinical or research support for study described, Stryker Spine. Mummaneni: consultant for DePuy Spine, Globus, and Stryker; direct stock ownership in Spinicity/ISD and Globus; clinical/research support for this study from NREF; royalties from DePuy Spine, Thieme Publishers, and Springer Publishers; grant from AOSpine; and honoraria from Globus.

[a] Department of Neurosurgery, University of California, San Francisco, 505 Parnassus Avenue, Room M779, San Francisco, CA 94143-0112, USA; [b] Department of Neurosurgery, Weill Cornell Medical College, 525 East 68th Street, Box 99, New York, NY 10065, USA; [c] Department of Neurosurgery, University of Michigan, 1500 East Medical Center Drive, SPC 5338, Ann Arbor, MI 48109-5338, USA
* Corresponding author.
E-mail address: praveen.mummaneni@ucsf.edu

Neurosurg Clin N Am 29 (2018) 399–406
https://doi.org/10.1016/j.nec.2018.03.007
1042-3680/18/© 2018 Elsevier Inc. All rights reserved.

increasingly elderly patient population with more concomitant medical comorbidities that is affected by lumbar deformity.

Not all patients with ASD are candidates for MIS correction. With the limited exposure inherent to MIS techniques, the MIS approaches may not be appropriate or optimal for severe and rigid deformities, especially in the sagittal plane. Previous studies have suggested that MIS approaches may undercorrect sagittal deformity in some cases.[15–18] Patient selection is critical but remains controversial in MIS for deformity correction. The minimally invasive spinal deformity surgery (MISDEF) algorithm was created to help guide surgeons in identifying which patients are candidates for deformity correction by MIS techniques (**Fig. 1**).[19] This article describes the modified MISDEF algorithm and presents representative cases.

MINIMALLY INVASIVE SPINAL DEFORMITY SURGERY DESIGN

The goals of treatment of ASD are decompression of neural elements, restoration of global coronal and sagittal alignment, and achievement of solid fusion. Numerous classification schemes have been proposed to guide the management of

ASD. In 2010, Silva and Lenke[20] published six levels of operative treatment (I-VI) to guide correction of ASD. The approach was based on several radiographic and clinical factors including presence of neurogenic claudication and radiculopathy, back pain, anterior osteophytes, olisthesis, coronal Cobb angle, lumbar kyphosis, and sagittal alignment. Based on these metrics, the authors recommended six different treatment levels of increasing complexity including decompression, posterior spinal fusion with instrumentation, anterior fusion, and osteotomies. These levels of treatment were meant to guide the surgeon in deciding the optimal open surgical approach to treat a patient's unique spinal pathology.

In recent years, spinopelvic alignment has been shown to be correlated with the impact of deformity on clinical health status and outcomes. To achieve optimal outcomes, a pelvic tilt (PT) less than 20°, pelvic incidence to lumbar lordosis mismatch (PI-LL) less than 10°, and sagittal vertical axis (SVA) less than 5 cm has been proposed. In accordance with these spinopelvic parameters, Mummaneni and colleagues[19] proposed the MISDEF algorithm (see **Fig. 1**) to provide a systematic guideline for surgeons to identify appropriate patients for a MIS approach for ASD

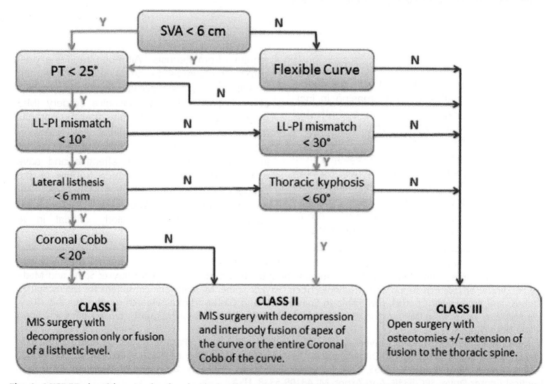

Fig. 1. MISDEF algorithm. LL, lumbar lordosis; N, no; PI, pelvic incidence; PT, pelvic tilt; SVA, sagittal vertical axis; Y, yes. (*From* Mummaneni PV, Shaffrey CI, Lenke LG, et al. The minimally invasive spinal deformity surgery algorithm: a reproducible rational framework for decision making in minimally invasive spinal deformity surgery. Neurosurg Focus 2014;36(5):E6; with permission.)

correction. The MISDEF algorithm was developed using the Delphi approach to gain agreement from experts in the field. This framework was created for adult patients with symptomatic deformity who have failed nonoperative therapies. The optimal approach is dependent on preoperative radiographic parameters. Based on these criteria, the appropriate surgical options range from MIS to traditional open techniques. The initial draft of this algorithm had six potential treatments but was found to have low interobserver and intraobserver reliability.

To simplify the algorithm and address this limitation, the authors redesigned the original algorithm to three general treatment-based classes. The class I approach included decompression alone or fusion of one listhetic level by a muscle-sparing MIS approach, either using a static or expandable tubular retractor. In class I cases, instrumentation is placed percutaneously or through the expandable tubular retractor. The class II approach comprises decompression and fusion via a multilevel MIS technique typically including the curve apex of the major curve. The class III approach is the traditional open approach with possible osteotomies or extension of fusion into the thoracic region.

To evaluate the reliability of this algorithm, 20 representative ASD cases were provided to 11 fellowship-trained spine surgeons for 2 rounds of assessments at least 2 months apart. These comprised 3, 10, and 7 MISDEF class I, II, and III patients, respectively. Clinical vignettes and preoperative standing scoliosis films were included. Interobserver kappa was 0.58 and 0.69 in the first and second rounds, respectively, and intraobserver kappa was 0.86, demonstrating substantial algorithm reproducibility and agreement among different surgeons.[19]

MINIMALLY INVASIVE SPINAL DEFORMITY SURGERY ALGORITHM

Several radiographic factors are considered in progressing through the MISDEF algorithm. Branch points are based on key spinopelvic parameters. These parameters include SVA, PT, PI-LL, lateral listhesis, and coronal Cobb angle. Previous investigations have highlighted the importance of these radiographic measures in influencing disability and outcome in patients with ASD. In a multicenter review of 752 patients with ASD, Glassman and colleagues[1] noted that increase in SVA linearly correlated with poorer scores several health care–related quality of life measures including the Scoliosis Research Society patient questionnaire, Oswestry Disability

Index (ODI), and Medical Outcomes Study 12-Item Short form. In a similar review of 73 adults with scoliosis, Mac-Thiong and coworkers[21] identified an association between SVA greater than 6 cm and worse disability (ODI >34).

Mismatch between PI and LL greater than 10° also correlates with worse disability. In a study of 492 patients with ASD, key spinopelvic parameters associated with worse health-related quality of life, defined by ODI greater than 40, was PT greater than or equal to 20°, SVA greater than or equal to 47 mm, and PI -LL greater than or equal to 11°.[22] Even in compensated spinopelvic deformity where SVA is normal, PI-LL is associated with worse disability.[23] In another study of 104 patients, Than and colleagues[24] compared the radiographic measures between patients with the "best" versus "worst" outcomes following MIS for ASD. The top 20% of patients based on change in ODI score ("best" group) were compared with the bottom 20% ("worst" group). Although there was no difference in preoperative PI-LL mismatch between these two groups, the best group had significantly less postoperative SVA (3.4 vs 6.9 cm) and PI-LL mismatch (10.4 vs 19.4°). Additionally, the best group had better outcomes on Visual Analog Scale scores for back and leg pain.

Given the reported importance of these spinopelvic parameters, the MISDEF algorithm is based on the preoperative radiographic evaluation using standing scoliosis radiographs. In addition, because of the reliance of first-generation MIS techniques on interbody fusion techniques that allow limited sagittal correction, patients with significant sagittal plane deformity are relegated to traditional open surgeries. Therefore, in cases of SVA less than 6 cm, the MISDEF algorithm guides surgeons toward class I and class II, favoring a MIS approach. However, if SVA is 7 or greater and the deformity is rigid, the algorithm tracks toward class III. Similarly, the degree of PI-LL mismatch and PT factor into whether a class III case is favored. Overall, milder deformity results in lower MISDEF class, favoring MIS techniques.

Class I

In general, patients with class I deformities present with neurogenic claudication or radiculopathy caused by stenosis of either the spinal canal, lateral recess, or foramina. Class I treatment includes MIS decompression with or without fusion at a single level. The patients who are candidates for class I treatment typically have an SVA less than 6 cm, PT less than 25°, LL-PI mismatch less than 10°, lateral listhesis of less than 6 mm, coronal Cobb angle of less than 20°, and thoracic kyphosis less than 60°. The goal of class I approach is decompression of the central canal or foraminal nerve roots at the lateral recess or foramina rather than correction of the sagittal or coronal alignment. MIS techniques are well suited in these cases, and decompression is achieved through a fixed or expandable tubular retractor. If indicated, as in a spondylolisthesis, a fusion can also be performed. Typically, this is either a MIS transforaminal lumbar interbody fusion (TLIF) or lateral lumbar interbody fusion (LLIF) with percutaneous instrumentation.

Class II

In addition to symptoms arising from stenosis, patients with class II deformities often present with more significant back pain associated with the deformity. These patients have SVA less than 6 cm, PI-LL 10° to 30°, major curve with coronal Cobb angle greater than 20°, and grade 1 or 2 spondylolisthesis or lateral listhesis. This class also comprises patients with SVA greater than or equal to 6 cm with flexible curves partially corrected in supine positioning. Similar to the surgical approach for class I patients, decompression is achieved by MIS through fixed or expandable tubular retractors at multiple levels. The surgeon can use multilevel MIS TLIF or LLIF in conjunction with percutaneous instrumentation. In contrast to class I, class II deformities require fusion at more than 1 level and may extend over the apex or the coronal Cobb angle of the major curve. This allows

for some correction of the deformity in addition to decompression.

Class III

Class III deformities often present with significant back and/or leg pain. These patients are characterized by a rigid curve and SVA greater than or equal to 6 cm, PI-LL greater than 30°, PT greater than 25°, and thoracic kyphosis greater than 60°. Patients within this class are not candidates for MIS. These significant deformities require traditional open surgery either with multilevel facet osteotomies or three-column osteotomies for more reliable correction of spinal alignment.

CASE EXAMPLES
Class I

This is a 72-year-old woman with isolated low back pain radiating into her right lateral leg and foot (**Fig. 2**). Imaging shows severe central and moderate neuroforaminal stenosis at L3-4 and lateral listhesis at L4-5. Patient was not fused and without prior instrumentation. Her spinal parameters were: SVA +2.6 cm, coronal Cobb 11°, LL 39°, PI 41°, PI-LL 2°, PT 14°, and sacral slope 27°. She underwent a right L3-4-5 hemilaminectomies, medial facetectomies, and foraminotomies.

Class II

This is a 64-year-old woman with history of a prior L5-S1 anterior/posterior fusion who developed

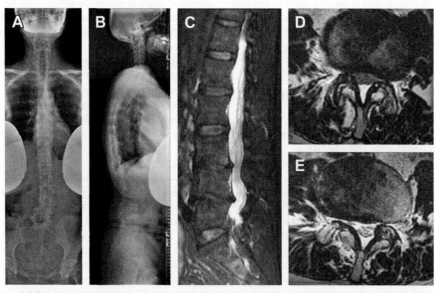

Fig. 2. Coronal (*A*) and sagittal (*B*) 36-inch standing radiographs showing convex left curvature of the lumbar spine. Preoperative T2-weighted sagittal (*C*) and axial MRI at L3-4 (*D*) and L4-5 (*E*) showing central and foraminal stenosis.

low back pain and left lower extremity radiculopathy (**Fig. 3**). MRI revealed multilevel foraminal stenosis. Her spinal parameters were SVA less than 1 cm, lumbar Cobb 34° with apex at L2, thoracic Cobb 49° with apex at T8, LL 53°, PI 64°, PI-LL 11°, PT 24°, and sacral slope 40°. She underwent L2-3, L3-4, L4-5 extreme lateral interbody fusions followed by minimally invasive posterior L2-S1 fixation. Her parameters improved to lumbar Cobb 21°, LL 61°, PI 64°, and PI-LL 3°.

Class III

This is a 65-year-old woman with a history of several prior lumbar fusions who presented with low back pain radiating into her left leg (**Fig. 4**). Imaging showed stenosis at L1-3 above her fusion with lumbar flat back and L2-3 spondylolisthesis. Her spinal parameters were SVA +9.0 cm, LL 33°, PI 54°, PI-LL 21°, PT 20°, and sacral slope 34°. She underwent a revision T11-pelvis fixation, L2-3 transforaminal lumbar interbody fusion, and L3 pedicle subtraction osteotomy. Postoperative spinal parameters were SVA +1.8 cm, LL 54°, PI 54°, PI-LL 0°.

FUTURE DIRECTIONS

One concern for MIS techniques, which mainly comprised LLIF or MIS TLIF at multiple levels with percutaneous fixation, was limited degree of sagittal correction. The original MISDEF algorithm was created to reflect the available techniques at the time of publication. Addressing the concern that early MIS techniques may not provide sufficient sagittal correction in cases of significant spinopelvic malalignment, the MISDEF algorithm was created to identify patients in which MIS was a reasonable option. Since the publication of the MISDEF algorithm in 2014, there have been advancements in MIS techniques and devices including anterior column release and new devices, such as hyperlordotic cages. Anterior column realignment is a more recent MIS technique that involves a lateral trans-psoas approach for discectomy and release of the anterior longitudinal ligament.[25,26] Lordotic interbody cages are placed and fixed to the vertebral bodies to lengthen the anterior column, and allow for an MIS approach to significantly improve sagittal alignment.

A revised MISDEF algorithm has been proposed to reflect contemporary MIS techniques and implant technology that have allowed for improved degree of sagittal correction (**Fig. 5**). The revised algorithm was designed via a modified Delphi technique and recommends four treatment classes that incorporate newer MIS

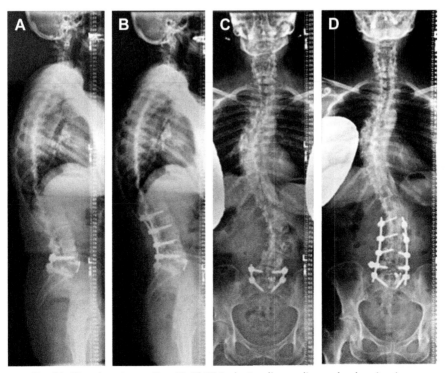

Fig. 3. Preoperative (*A, C*) and postoperative (*B, D*) 36-inch standing radiographs showing improvement in the spinal parameters.

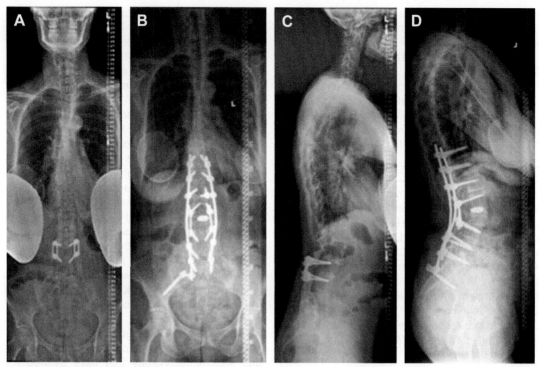

Fig. 4. Preoperative (*A, C*) and postoperative (*B, D*) 36-inch standing radiographs showing improvement in lumbar lordosis and sagittal alignment.

approaches. Similar to the original, the revised algorithm is based on the radiographic parameters: SVA, PT, LL-PI mismatch, and coronal Cobb. Additionally, the algorithm considers whether the spine is rigid, the extent of fusion needed, and pre-existing multilevel instrumentation. Reliability of this algorithm is currently being evaluated.

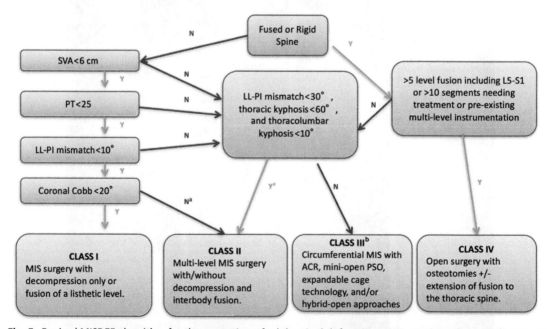

Fig. 5. Revised MISDEF algorithm for the correction of adult spinal deformity. ACR, anterior column realignment; N, no; PSO, pedicle subtraction osteotomy; Y, yes. [a] For curved greater than 60, double major curves, consider class III. [b] For experienced MIS surgeons.

SUMMARY

Appropriate patient selection using the MISDEF algorithm can help guide surgeons in identifying candidates for MIS in deformity correction. The algorithm, which has been shown to be reliable and reproducible, is based on key radiographic parameters: SVA, PI-LL mismatch, PT, and coronal Cobb angle. These metrics guide surgeons toward three treatment classes. Because the algorithm focuses only on radiographic measures of deformity, clinical features including symptomatology and medical comorbidities should be taken into account. Future studies will aim to validate the MISDEF algorithm and its impact on postoperative outcomes.

REFERENCES

1. Glassman SD, Bridwell K, Dimar JR, et al. The impact of positive sagittal balance in adult spinal deformity. Spine (Phila Pa 1976) 2005;30(18): 2024–9.

2. Schwab F, Dubey A, Gamez L, et al. Adult scoliosis: prevalence, SF-36, and nutritional parameters in an elderly volunteer population. Spine (Phila Pa 1976) 2005;30(9):1082–5.

3. Schwab F, Dubey A, Pagala M, et al. Adult scoliosis: a health assessment analysis by SF-36. Spine (Phila Pa 1976) 2003;28(6):602–6.

4. Schwab F, Farcy JP, Bridwell K, et al. A clinical impact classification of scoliosis in the adult. Spine (Phila Pa 1976) 2006;31(18):2109–14.

5. Daffner SD, Vaccaro AR. Adult degenerative lumbar scoliosis. Am J Orthop (Belle Mead NJ) 2003;32(2): 77–82 [discussion: 82].

6. Winter RB, Lonstein JE, Denis F. Pain patterns in adult scoliosis. Orthop Clin North Am 1988;19(2): 339–45.

7. Smith JS, Shaffrey CI, Berven S, et al. Improvement of back pain with operative and nonoperative treatment in adults with scoliosis. Neurosurgery 2009; 65(1):86–93 [discussion: 93–4].

8. Smith JS, Shaffrey CI, Berven S, et al. Operative versus nonoperative treatment of leg pain in adults with scoliosis: a retrospective review of a prospective multicenter database with two-year follow-up. Spine (Phila Pa 1976) 2009;34(16):1693–8.

9. Dhall SS, Wang MY, Mummaneni PV. Clinical and radiographic comparison of mini-open transforaminal lumbar interbody fusion with open transforaminal lumbar interbody fusion in 42 patients with long-term follow-up. J Neurosurg Spine 2008;9(6): 560–5.

10. Foley KT, Gupta SK. Percutaneous pedicle screw fixation of the lumbar spine: preliminary clinical results. J Neurosurg 2002;97(1 Suppl):7–12.

11. Guiot BH, Khoo LT, Fessler RG. A minimally invasive technique for decompression of the lumbar spine. Spine (Phila Pa 1976) 2002;27(4):432–8.

12. Scheufler KM. Technique and clinical results of minimally invasive reconstruction and stabilization of the thoracic and thoracolumbar spine with expandable cages and ventrolateral plate fixation. Neurosurgery 2007;61(4):798–808 [discussion: 808–9].

13. Anand N, Baron EM, Thaiyananthan G, et al. Minimally invasive multilevel percutaneous correction and fusion for adult lumbar degenerative scoliosis: a technique and feasibility study. J Spinal Disord Tech 2008;21(7):459–67.

14. Benglis DM, Elhammady MS, Levi AD, et al. Minimally invasive anterolateral approaches for the treatment of back pain and adult degenerative deformity. Neurosurgery 2008;63(3 Suppl):191–6.

15. Wang MY, Mummaneni PV. Minimally invasive surgery for thoracolumbar spinal deformity: initial clinical experience with clinical and radiographic outcomes. Neurosurg Focus 2010;28(3):E9.

16. Tormenti MJ, Maserati MB, Bonfield CM, et al. Complications and radiographic correction in adult scoliosis following combined transpsoas extreme lateral interbody fusion and posterior pedicle screw instrumentation. Neurosurg Focus 2010;28(3):E7.

17. Anand N, Rosemann R, Khalsa B, et al. Mid-term to long-term clinical and functional outcomes of minimally invasive correction and fusion for adults with scoliosis. Neurosurg Focus 2010;28(3):E6.

18. Dakwar E, Cardona RF, Smith DA, et al. Early outcomes and safety of the minimally invasive, lateral retroperitoneal transpsoas approach for adult degenerative scoliosis. Neurosurg Focus 2010;28(3):E8.

19. Mummaneni PV, Shaffrey CI, Lenke LG, et al. The minimally invasive spinal deformity surgery algorithm: a reproducible rational framework for decision making in minimally invasive spinal deformity surgery. Neurosurg Focus 2014;36(5):E6.

20. Silva FE, Lenke LG. Adult degenerative scoliosis: evaluation and management. Neurosurg Focus 2010;28(3):E1.

21. Mac-Thiong JM, Transfeldt EE, Mehbod AA, et al. Can c7 plumbline and gravity line predict health related quality of life in adult scoliosis? Spine (Phila Pa 1976) 2009;34(15):E519–27.

22. Schwab FJ, Blondel B, Bess S, et al. Radiographical spinopelvic parameters and disability in the setting of adult spinal deformity: a prospective multicenter analysis. Spine (Phila Pa 1976) 2013;38(13):E803–12.

23. Smith JS, Singh M, Klineberg E, et al. Surgical treatment of pathological loss of lumbar lordosis (flatback) in patients with normal sagittal vertical axis achieves similar clinical improvement as surgical treatment of elevated sagittal vertical axis: clinical article. J Neurosurg Spine 2014;21(2):160–70.

24. Than KD, Park P, Fu KM, et al. Clinical and radiographic parameters associated with best versus worst clinical outcomes in minimally invasive spinal deformity surgery. J Neurosurg Spine 2016;25(1): 21–5.

25. Saigal R, Mundis GM Jr, Eastlack R, et al. Anterior column realignment (ACR) in adult sagittal deformity correction: technique and review of the literature. Spine (Phila Pa 1976) 2016;41(Suppl 8):S66–73.

26. Akbarnia BA, Mundis GM Jr, Moazzaz P, et al. Anterior column realignment (ACR) for focal kyphotic spinal deformity using a lateral transpsoas approach and ALL release. J Spinal Disord Tech 2014;27(1): 29–39.

Transpsoas Approach Nuances

Randall J. Hlubek, MD[a,b,c], Robert K. Eastlack, MD[a,b], Gregory M. Mundis Jr, MD[a,b,*]

KEYWORDS

- Lateral lumbar interbody fusion • Transpsoas approach • Adult spinal deformity
- Degenerative spine

KEY POINTS

- The transpsoas approach requires meticulous preoperative planning to optimize safety and achieve operative alignment goals.
- Once the dilator is expanded within the psoas, the operation must be performed in a maximally efficient manner to minimize neural injury.
- In order to maximize sagittal plane correction, a posterior approach with posterior column osteotomies may be required.

INTRODUCTION

Adult spinal deformity (ASD) secondary to the degenerative process is a potentially debilitating condition with a substantially negative impact on function and quality of life.[1] As the population continues to age,[2] the number of patients requiring treatment of degenerative deformity will certainly increase. Although operative treatment has been shown to result in significant improvement in health-related quality-of-life measures,[3,4] risks associated with surgical correction are substantial. Mitigating these risks is crucial in optimizing the risk/benefit ratio in this predominantly elderly population.

Traditional open posterior approaches are considered the gold standard for deformity correction, but this technique is associated with high rates of surgical morbidity.[5,6] Although the open approach may be necessary in patients with severe sagittal imbalance and/or rigid deformities,[7,8] the transpsoas approach offers a minimally invasive tissue-sparing corridor to the spine that allows for anterior column reconstruction and fusion with potentially less blood loss and morbidity. Phillips and colleagues[9] demonstrated that restoration of disc height with the transpsoas lateral lumbar interbody fusion (LLIF) is safe and effective for correcting coronal deformities in patients with ASD.

Although coronal alignment is an important component of ASD surgery, restoration of sagittal balance is a priority when reconstructing the spine.[10,11] There are concerns regarding the ability of the LLIF alone to restore sagittal balance in cases of moderate/severe malalignment.[8,12] To optimize segmental lordosis and sagittal plane correction, hybrid approaches involving LLIF and open posterior column osteotomies have been used with significant improvements in sagittal alignment.[13–15] Further evolution of this technique has involved anterior column realignment (ACR)

Disclosure Statement: Dr R.J. Hlubek: no disclosures. Dr G.M. Mundis: consultant for NuVasive and K2M. Dr R.K. Eastlack: consultant for NuVasive, Alphatec, Seaspine, Aesculap, and Titan; ownership in NuVasive; direct stock ownership in Alphatec and Seaspine; and patent holder with Globus Medical, Titan, NuTech, Invuity, and Spine Innovation.

[a] Department of Orthopedics, Scripps Clinic, 10666 North Torrey Pines Road, La Jolla, CA 92037, USA; [b] San Diego Center for Spinal Disorders, 6190 Cornerstone, San Diego, CA 92121, USA; [c] Division of Neurosurgery, Barrow Neurological Institute, 350 W Thomas Road, Phoenix, AZ 85013, USA
* Corresponding author. San Diego Spine Foundation, 6190 Cornerstone Court Suite 212, San Diego, CA 92121.
E-mail address: Gmundis1@gmail.com

with sectioning of the anterior longitudinal ligament (ALL) and placement of hyperlordotic interbody grafts.[16,17] ACR can provide sagittal plane correction similar to that of a pedicle subtraction osteotomy (PSO).[18] Thus, the transpsoas approach is a powerful tool in correcting sagittal deformity but may require posterior column osteotomies and/or anterior longitudinal ligament release to achieve spinal alignment goals. The purpose of this article is to evaluate the use of the transpsoas approach in correcting adult spinal deformity.

INDICATIONS/CONTRAINDICATIONS

Approach selection is imperative to obtaining optimal results in patients with ASD. The minimally invasive spinal deformity surgery (MISDEF) algorithm was created to provide a framework for decision-making. Patients are divided into 3 classes based on radiographic characteristics and treatment plans. Class I (sagittal vertical axis [SVA] <6 cm, pelvic tilt [PT] < 25°, PI-LL mismatch <10°, cobb angle <20°) and class II (SVA >6 cm, PT <25°, Pelvic incidence minus lumbar lordosis (PI-LL) mismatch <30°, cobb angle >20°) patients are amendable to Minimally invasive spine techniques. Class III patients (SVA >6 cm, PT >25°, PI-LL mismatch >30°, cobb angle >20°) represent severe coronal and/or sagittal malalignment and typically require open surgery to adequately correct the alignment.[7]

Table 1 provides a list of indications/contraindications for the transpsoas approach in patients with ASD. The indications for LLIF are vast and may be used in patients with class I and II ASD as a stand-alone construct or in combination with other techniques. Relative contraindications include prior retroperitoneal surgery, fused operative levels, and unfavorable neurovascular anatomy that would prevent safe access to the operative levels.

PREOPERATIVE PLANNING
Alignment

Anteroposterior (AP) and lateral full-length 36-in radiographs should be performed to evaluate the extent of the deformity and to plan the correction. If available, whole-body EOS imaging (Paris, France) should be obtained to ascertain true global alignment. The 3 radiographic parameters with the strongest correlations with disability are PT, SVA, and PI-LL mismatch.[19] The goals of surgery are to obtain a PT of less than 20°, an SVA of 5 cm or less, and a PI-LL mismatch within 10°. The T1 pelvic angle is a radiographic parameter of global spinopelvic alignment that accounts for sagittal alignment and PT with a single measurement and ideally should be less than 20°.[20] Recent literature supports the notion that total body sagittal alignment (head to ankles) is a better predictor of outcomes in patients with ASD. Kim and colleagues[21] described the cranial SVA as a measure of total body alignment and found that it is a stronger predictor of clinical outcomes than the C7 SVA in patients with adult deformity. Another critical development in our understanding of ASD is that operative realignment targets should account for age, with elderly patients requiring different realignment goals than their younger counterparts.[22]

Understanding the degree of correction that can be achieved with the transpsoas approach is critical to achieving these goals. Segmental correction will vary with cage size/lordotic angle and release of the spine with anterior column realignment/ALL sectioning and/or posterior column osteotomies (**Table 2**). The degree of sagittal correction also depends on the level being addressed and the native segmental alignment typically appreciated by that level. Uribe and colleagues[23] measured the effect of varying lordotic cages and ALL release on segmental lordosis, although their study did not assess these changes by individual lumbar segment. In that study, a 10°

Table 1
Indications/contraindications for the transpsoas approach in patients with adult spinal deformity

Indications	Contraindications
MISDEF class I, II	Fusion at the operative levels
Restoration of disc height	Prior retroperitoneal surgery
Indirect decompression	Ventral location of the lumbar plexus
Anterior column realignment	MISDEF class III

Table 2
Segmental correction

Implant Lordosis (°)	ALL Release	Posterior Column Osteotomy	Degree of Correction (°)
10	N	N	0.9
10	Y	N	4.1
20	Y	N	9.5
30	Y	N	11.6
20, 30	Y	Y	19.9

implant with an intact ALL provided an average of a 0.9° increase in segmental lordosis. With the addition of ALL release in the setting of 10°, 20°, 30° implants, the resultant segmental lordosis was 4.1°, 9.5°, and 11.6°, respectively. The failure to achieve as much segmental lordosis as the lateral implants, even with an ALL release, is related to constraint of the posterior elements as well as the native pliability of residual annular and ligamentous tissue that varies by level and individual. The addition of posterior column osteotomies to ALL release leads to an average increase of 19° of lordosis.[24]

Assessment of the preoperative coronal alignment is important in order to prevent postoperative coronal imbalance. Bao and colleagues[25] described 3 different types of coronal alignment. If the coronal offset between the C7 plumb line and the central sacral vertical line was less than 3 cm it was considered a type A curve. Type B and C curves had coronal offsets greater than 3 cm toward the concavity and convexity of the curve respectively. Type C curves were at greatest risk of postoperative coronal malalignment and were typically secondary to undercorrection of

the fractional curve (FC). The coronal FC typically occurs below (most often L4-S1) the major curve in the midlumbar spine and is a common finding in patients with coronal deformities. Correction of the FC should be considered during surgical planning and may require treatment with a supplemental or alternative approach (**Fig. 1**).

MRI of the Lumbar Spine

MRI provides information regarding the degree and location of neural compression. Although several studies have reported the efficacy of LLIF for indirect decompression of the foramen,[26,27] the effects on central and lateral recess stenosis are not as clear. Ligamentous central stenosis may be indirectly decompressed with LLIF because of the restoration of the disc height and stretching of the posterior longitudinal ligament and ligamentum flavum.[28] However, direct decompression may be necessary in cases of severe central stenosis secondary to facet/bony hypertrophy.

Location of the lumbar plexus and retroperitoneal vessels should be carefully studied. Patients

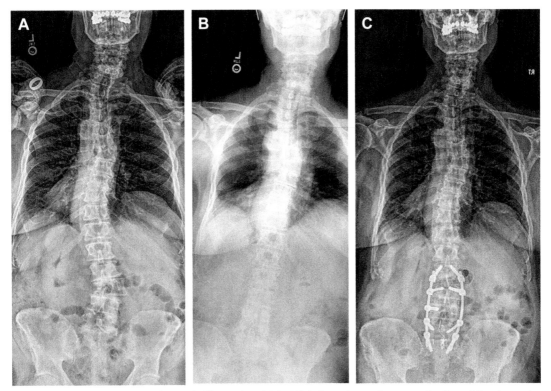

Fig. 1. (*A*) Preoperative AP radiograph illustrating L4-S1 FC below the major curve in the midlumbar spine. (*B*) Postoperative AP radiograph illustrating coronal malalignment following an L2-5 LLIF with inadequate correction of the FC. (*C*) Postoperative AP radiograph with restoration of coronal balance following correction of the FC with an L5-S1 Anterior lumbar interbody fusion (ALIF) and L2-S1 pedicle screw fixation.

with ASD have altered locations of their neurovascular structures, which result in the reduction of the safe surgical corridor for the transpsoas approach.[29] Psoas morphology and location should be analyzed, especially at L4-5. Anterior versus lateral positioning of the psoas muscle relative to the disc space is associated with anterior migration of the lumbar plexus and posterolateral migration of the iliac vasculature.[30,31]

Approach Side

Coronal imaging should be analyzed to determine if the angle of approach to the L4-5 disc space will be too substantial as a result of the iliac crest. With coronal deformities, often one side will provide favorable access to the L4-5 disc space as a result of its coronal tilt, whereas access on the contralateral side will be challenging or impossible because of the iliac crest. The coronal L4-5 disc angle is typically more accessible from the concave side of the primary lumbar deformity.

Approaching from the concavity of the scoliotic curve is favorable for several reasons. Placing patients with the convex portion of the curve on the operative table provides some correction of the coronal deformity with positioning and gentle breaking of the table. This correction facilitates the correction achieved with LLIF. Trajectories through the disc spaces of lumbar curves will converge on the concave side often allowing for a single skin and fascial incision, in many cases, whereas multiple incisions may be required on the convex side. Additionally, the most collapsed and contracted portion of the disc space, and the most severe foraminal stenosis, is on the concave side. Theoretically, releasing the deformity and restoring disc height from the concave side may lead to improved correction of the deformity and greater indirect decompression of the foramen.

PREPARATION AND PATIENT POSITIONING

Before positioning patients, the operating room table should be evaluated to ensure that there are no obstructions to obtaining AP and lateral radiographs with the C-arm. Patients are then placed in the lateral decubitus position with the approach side facing up. The iliac crest should be placed at the break of the bed with the hips at approximately 30° of flexion and knees in 90° of flexion to reduce tension on the psoas and lumbar plexus.[27] A roll is placed in the axilla to prevent brachial plexus injury and all pressure points are adequately padded. To restrict movement and rotation of patients on the operative table, rolls may be placed on the ventral and dorsal aspect of patients' thoracolumbar (TL)

region. The iliac crest and chest is then secured to the bed with tape in a fashion that does not inhibit the ability of the table to break. With more severe rotational deformities, provisional taping at the pelvis/hips with imaging assessment of the full spectrum of table rotation required to achieve AP views of all surgical segments is encouraged. The iliac crest is then pulled inferiorly with tape that spans the hip and legs. If necessary, although not commonly performed, flexing the table at the break will open the space between the 12th rib and iliac crest, and thus enhance access to the L4-5 disc space. This can provide some correction of the deformity, as well. However, this should only be done to the extent necessary, since this maneuver increases tension on the psoas and lumbar plexus.[31] A true AP and lateral radiograph is then obtained for the initial LLIF level. Table adjustments with Trendelenburg and reverse Trendelenburg maneuvers will assist in obtaining a true lateral radiograph, whereas adjustments with rotation of the bed will alter the AP radiograph. The wigwag of the C-arm should be adjusted to match the angle of the disc space. Because of the segmental 3-dimensional deformity that is often present in patients with ASD, each operative level will require unique table adjustments to obtain a true AP and lateral radiograph.

SURGICAL APPROACH

Either a single-incision[32] or a 2-incision[33] technique may be used to access the retroperitoneal space. For the 2-incision technique, the additional incision is placed along the lateral border of the erector spinae muscles between the crest and 12th rib. The additional incision allows for blunt dissection into the retroperitoneal space and mobilization of peritoneum off the psoas and facilitates the passage of dilators/retractors. These objectives can be accomplished with a single-incision technique as well. However, the 2-incision technique may be advantageous in approaching the TL junction, as it assists with mobilization of the diaphragm and connection of the retro-pleural and retroperitoneal spaces.

In cases that require multilevel lateral fusions, thoughtful consideration regarding the sequence of operative levels is important. Typically, L4-5 should be the initial operative level for several reasons. The location of the lumbar plexus at this level may prohibit safe access to the disc space, and the approach may have to be aborted. If this level is inaccessible, then a different approach altogether may be necessary for the treatment of the deformity. The next level that should be performed is the most cranial level (when it resides in the TL junction [T11-L2]). If the caudal levels are sequentially performed before the TL junction levels, as the spine straightens out the angles and access to this region will become less favorable through a single incision below the diaphragm.

A detailed understanding of the lumbar plexus anatomy within the retroperitoneum and abdominal wall musculature is critical to preventing neurologic injury during the early stages of the approach. Dakwar and colleagues[34] performed cadaveric dissections to describe the branches of the lumbar plexus outside the psoas muscle. The 4 main nerves that travel outside the psoas are the subcostal, iliohypogastric, ilioinguinal, and lateral femoral cutaneous nerves. The subcostal nerve originates from the T12 root and has both motor and sensory components. It travels along the inferior border of the 12th rib before coursing anterior to the upper portion of the quadratus lumborum. It then penetrates the transversalis fascia and supplies the abdominal musculature especially the external oblique muscles. The iliohypogastric and ilioinguinal nerves have motor and sensory components and arise from the T12-L1 and L1 nerves, respectively. They emerge from the upper lateral portion of the psoas muscle and run obliquely through the retroperitoneal space before piercing the abdominal wall musculature and supplying the transversus abdominis and internal oblique muscles. The lateral femoral cutaneous nerve is purely sensory and arises from L2-L3. It emerges from the lateral border of the psoas at the L4 level and travels obliquely across the iliacus muscle. The nerve then continues through or below the inguinal ligament approximately 1 cm medial to the anterior superior iliac spine. Injury to these nerves may result in abdominal wall paresis and sensory deficits along the corresponding dermatome.

Once the incision centered over the operative levels is made, blunt dissection is carried down to the superficial muscle fascia. This layer is then dissected along the length of the skin incision. Care must be taken to avoid injury to the iliohypogastric and ilioinguinal nerves, and electrocautery should be avoided to prevent thermal injury to the nerves. Dissection through the external oblique, internal oblique, and transversalis abdominis muscles is carried out along the direction of the muscle fibers. If a nerve branch is encountered, it is dissected and mobilized away from the approach. The transversalis fascia is then penetrated and the retroperitoneal space is entered. The index finger is then used to identify relevant landmarks. The transverse process is easily palpated, and the psoas muscle can be located directly medial and the quadratus lumborum

posterolateral. The lateral border of the psoas is then swept to ensure the peritoneum is clear from injury with the dilators. Care must be taken to not injure traversing retroperitoneal nerves (lateral femoral cutaneous) by mistaking them for adhesions.

After the psoas muscle has been identified and surrounding tissue swept free, the next step is to place the initial dilator through the psoas and on to the disc space. Knowledge of the lumbar plexus anatomy within the psoas is important in understanding the safe working zones. In a cadaveric study, Uribe and colleagues[35] defined the anatomic safe zones relative to the disc spaces at each level. The area between the anterior and posterior border of the vertebral body was divided into the 4 following zones: zone I (anterior quarter), zone II (middle anterior quarter), zone III (posterior middle quarter), and zone IV (posterior quarter). The femoral nerve of the lumbar plexus (L2, L3, L4) is found deep within the psoas muscle and descends along the lumbar spine in a gradual posterior to anterior trajectory from zone IV at the L3-4 level and into zone III and IV at the L4-5 level. The genitofemoral nerve (L1-2) crosses the L2-3 disc space at zone II and courses anteriorly into zone I at L3-4 and L4-5. The safe corridors to prevent injury to the femoral and genitofemoral nerves were identified to be the middle posterior quarter (zone III) at the L1-4 levels and at the midpoint of the L4-5 level (zone II-III junction).

Directional dynamically triggered electromyography (t-EMG) mitigates the risk of neural injury during the approach by indicating both the direction and proximity of a nerve.[36,37] T-EMG is delivered to the distal end of the dilator as it is passed through the psoas. Direct nerve stimulation has been shown clinically to elicit average EMG responses of 2 mA.[38,39] Thresholds less than 5 mA indicate possible direct contact with the nerve. Perhaps more important than the threshold is the directionality of the threshold. Once the dilator is confirmed with lateral fluoroscopy to be at the appropriate safe zone, it is rotated 360° to elicit positional thresholds in all directions. Ideally, the lower thresholds should be in the posterior direction and higher thresholds should be in the anterior direction. This position would indicate that the femoral nerve is posterior to the dilator. If t-EMG indicates that the femoral nerve is anterior, then the dilator must be repositioned.

Once the dilator is in the appropriate position and t-EMG indicates the femoral nerve is posterior, then a Kirschner wire (K wire) is placed through the dilator and into the disc space. This may be challenging in patients with ASD with collapsed disc spaces along the concavity. If unable to gain access to the disc space with the K wire, the K wire may be carefully malleted into the osteophyte or bone adjacent to the disc space; subtle repositioning of the retractor can occur following its initial placement. After the series of tubular dilators are advanced through the psoas with t-EMG, the retractor is then placed and secured to the articulating arm. The K wire remains while the dilators are removed. Direct visual inspection and a manually triggered EMG probe are used to interrogate the field and to specifically ensure that there are no nerves along the posterior blade (where the intradiscal shim blade may be placed). If used, the intradiscal shim blade is then placed within the posterior blade. This placement ensures that this blade is locked into position while the other blades retract away from it.

The retractor expansion should be minimized to that required for discectomy and cage insertion in order to prevent unnecessary psoas trauma and neurologic injury. Once the retractor is opened, the rest of the operation must proceed as efficiently as possible. Uribe and colleagues[40] demonstrated that prolonged retraction time was a predictor of postoperative neuropraxia. In cases of prolonged retraction time, increasing t-EMG thresholds may indicate neural compromise and warrant removal of the retractor for a period to eliminate compression of the nerves.

SURGICAL PROCEDURE

All steps of this procedure should be performed with the instruments orthogonal to the floor to ensure that there are no injuries to the vascular structures ventrally or the spinal canal dorsally. Total retractor time should be limited to approximately 30 minutes per level. Uribe and colleagues[40] reported that retraction time was significantly longer in those patients with symptomatic neuropraxia versus those without (32.3 vs 22.6 minutes). If it seems that more time is needed, then the authors recommend collapsing the retractor for a period to theoretically limit the risk of ischemic injury to the neural structures.

- Step 1: A wide annulotomy is made with the knife in a rectangular fashion. It should ideally encompass the end plates, posterior to the ALL, and just anterior to the posterior blade. If an intradiscal shim is used posteriorly, a 1- to 2-mm of annular cuff should be preserved ventral to it, which prevents migration of the retractor in the anterior direction.
- Step 2: A Cobb elevator is then advanced down both the inferior and superior end plate.

If there is any resistance during this maneuver, AP fluoroscopy should be taken to ensure that the end plates are not being violated and that the trajectory is appropriate. This step is critical in preparation of the disc space. The Cobb is ideally passed subchondrally to delaminate the disc fully from the vertebral end plate efficiently. Once the contralateral side has been reached, the Cobb is gently malleted to release the contralateral annulus. This procedure is performed along both the inferior and superior end plates. Release of the contralateral annulus will facilitate correction of the deformity.

- Step 3: The pituitary rongeur is used to remove readily accessible disc material. This step should be efficient and only remove material that is free. The following steps will ensure the disc is appropriately prepared
- Step 4: The optional step of using a box chisel to debulk the disc space of disc more rapidly can be used now. Before malleting it into the disc space, AP fluoroscopy should be used to ensure the box cutter is orthogonal with the disc space. The horizontal portion of the T-handle should be oriented in the same direction as the disc space to mitigate the risk of end plate violation (**Fig. 2**).
- Step 5: Interbody trials are then placed into the disc space. AP fluoroscopy of the trial will assist with determining the optimal dimensions of the interbody. The height is determined by tactile feel and the degree of resistance required in removing the trial. Ensure that the trials complete the contralateral annular release/rupture, which is most easily accomplished with the initial and thinnest trial. Once the appropriate height is determined, lateral fluoroscopy confirms the position of the trial in the anteroposterior direction. It is not uncommon for distraction of severely degenerated disc spaces to result in ALL rupture. In cases whereby the ALL is inadvertently released or made incompetent, implants with integrated fixation should be considered to prevent migration of the implant.
- Step 6: Continue end plate preparation while the interbody cage and graft are being prepared. During step 6, the operating room technician is made aware of the length, width, height, and lordotic angles for the graft. While this graft is being prepared on the back table, rasps and stirrup curettes are used to remove residual cartilage and disc material from the end plates. Care must be taken to not violate the end plates with these instruments.

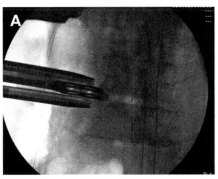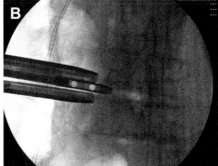

Fig. 2. (*A*) Intraoperative AP radiograph demonstrating nonorthogonal orientation of the box chisel with potential end plate violation. (*B*) Intraoperative AP radiograph demonstrating proper orthogonal orientation of the box chisel.

- *Step 7: The interbody graft is delivered.* Graft containment guides are used to guide the interbody into the disc space and prevent the egress of allograft from the interbody cage. The blades are removed and the interbody is advanced with a mallet into its final position. The retractor is removed while inspecting the surgical field for bleeding. Optionally, a small deep drain can be placed over the psoas to collect any blood that may collect and further irritate the retroperitoneal structures.

COMPLICATIONS AND MANAGEMENT

See **Table 3**.

- *Motor*: Transient hip flexor weakness is found in 24% of patients and is secondary to trauma to the psoas muscle during dissection and retraction.[41] Care should be taken to minimize retractor openings and duration during the operation. Motor weakness secondary to root or lumbar plexus injury is less common and occurs with an incidence of 4.5%.[40] Directional t-EMG decreases the risk of nerve injury during the approach providing the direction and proximity of the motor nerves. Indirect ischemic injury secondary to stretching or compression may occur with retraction. Limiting retraction time with efficient disc space preparation may reduce the incidence of neuropraxia. Symptomatic neuropraxia typically recovers within 3 months.[42]
- *Sensory*: Sensory nerves within the lumbar plexus are at risk during the operation, and t-EMG will not assist in their detection or localization. Lykissas and colleagues[43] reported postoperative sensory deficits in 38% of patients with complete resolution in most patients. Particularly vulnerable nerves including those located within the abdominal

wall (iliohypogastric, ilioinguinal), retroperitoneum (lateral femoral cutaneous nerve), and within the psoas (genitofemoral nerve). Knowledge of the course of these nerves and careful dissection will help prevent injury.

- *Abdominal wall paresis*: Injury to the motor component of the subcostal nerve, iliohypogastric, and/or ilioinguinal can lead to paresis and bulging of the abdominal musculature they innervate. Dakwar and colleagues[44] reported a 1.8% incidence of this complication with 80% of patients completely recovering

Table 3
Complications and prevention

Complication	Incidence (%)	Avoidance
Transient hip flexor weakness	24.0	Minimize retractor opening and duration
Lumbar plexus injury	4.5	Directional t-EMG
Sensory deficit	38.0	Careful dissection down to the psoas
Abdominal wall paresis	1.8	Careful dissection down to the psoas
Vessel injury	0.10	True AP/lateral radiographs and maintaining instruments orthogonal to the floor
Bowel injury	0.08	Mobilization of the peritoneum off the psoas
Subsidence	14.0	Avoidance of end plate violation

Table 4
Radiographic and clinical outcome data for relevant studies

Author	Approach	N	Levels	Operative Time (min)	Estimated Blood Loss (mL)	Cobb (°) Before	Cobb (°) After	PI-LL (°) Before	PI-LL (°) After	SVA (mm) Before	SVA (mm) After	PT (°) Before	PT (°) After	Major Complications (%)	ODI Before	ODI After
Wang et al,[13] 2014	Stand-alone	7	3.7	355	95	36	30	NA	NA	38	38	34	36	29	49	26
	Circumferential	43	4.3	479	585	32	12	NA	NA	29	30	26	25	14	43	23
	Hybrid	35	4.2	1743	1743	43	15	NA	NA	63	29	34	25	40	51	34
Strom et al,[14] 2016	Hybrid	32	10.0	404	1129	35	13	17	−5	65	37	22	20	NA	50	29
	Open only	60	11.0	304	1883	28	14	18	2	74	37	21	18	NA	51	39
Theologis et al,[15] 2017	Hybrid	16	11.0	859	2460	49	22	23	7	63	36	25	20	56	51	35
	Open only	16	9.0	379	1993	36	24	17	11	64	60	25	24	13	43	26

Abbreviations: NA, Not applicable; ODI, Oswestry Disability Index.

within 6 months. These nerves reside in the abdominal wall musculature, and careful dissection during the approach is necessary to prevent injury. Electrocautery should be avoided to eliminate the risk of thermal injury to these nerves.

- *Vessel injury*: Vascular injury should be rare with the transpsoas approach because the major vessels move more anteriorly in the lateral decubitus position. However, injury to the major vessels has been reported to occur with an incidence of 0.10%.[45] Packing with hemostatic agents or direct surgical repair are the treatment options. The key to avoiding this complication is ensuring that a true AP and lateral fluoroscopy at the operative level has been obtained. While performing the discectomy and end plate preparation, all instrumentation should be orthogonal to the floor. In all cases, hemostatic agents should be readily available should any bleeding occur. It is also critical to scrutinize the location of vascular structures, both ipsilaterally and contralaterally, during the planning of surgery; this will aid in avoiding injury to the vessels during approach or contralateral annular release.
- *Bowel injury*: The incidence of bowel injury is reported to be 0.08%.[45] Treatment typically consists of a laparotomy with washout, debridement, and diverting colostomy. The risk of this complication can be diminished with adequate mobilization of the peritoneum. Care should be taken to guide the dilators and retractor down to the psoas ensuring that the peritoneum is not entrapped. Patients with prior retroperitoneal surgery or radiation may have dense adhesions that do not allow for mobilization of the peritoneum. A safe transpsoas approach may not be feasible in this population.
- *Subsidence*: Le and colleagues[46] reported a 14% incidence of subsidence and found that construct length had a significant positive correlation with increased subsidence rates. There are several methods to decrease the risk of subsidence, including avoidance of end plate violation, ensuring the interbody graft spans the end plate apophysis, placing the widest graft possible, using supplemental fixation, and avoiding overstuffing of the disc space.

POSTOPERATIVE CARE

- Mobilization on the day of surgery
- Bracing for comfort
- Bowel care regimen

- AP and lateral full-length 36-in radiographs to evaluate global sagittal and coronal balance

OUTCOMES

Table 4 provides radiographic and clinical outcome data for relevant studies. These studies highlight the ability of the transpsoas approach to correct sagittal and coronal plane deformities. Stand-alone LLIF constructs or LLIF with percutaneous pedicle screw fixation may be appropriate in patients with minimal sagittal malalignment. However, in patients with moderate sagittal deformity, LLIF with posterior column osteotomies may be necessary to optimize sagittal correction. Although the clinical and radiographic outcomes of ACR are not discussed in this article, emerging evidence suggests that this transpsoas technique provides similar correction to PSO.[18] With the evolving ACR technique, patients with class III MISDEF or those with severe sagittal malalignment may potentially be treated with a transpsoas approach and percutaneous pedicle screw fixation.

SUMMARY

The transpsoas approach is a powerful tool in correcting ASD secondary to the degenerative process. It may be used as a stand-alone construct or in combination with other approaches to correct both coronal and sagittal malalignment. Preoperative planning with careful analysis of full-length 36-in radiographs and an MRI of the lumbar spine is essential in determining the safety and feasibility of this approach. Ultimately the goals of deformity correction must be achieved, and LLIF is a valuable tool that can aid in achieving these goals while minimizing perioperative morbidity.

REFERENCES

1. Glassman SD, Bridwell K, Dimar JR, et al. The impact of positive sagittal balance in adult spinal deformity. Spine (Phila Pa 1976) 2005;30:2024–9.
2. He W, Goodkind D, Kowal P. An aging world: 2015. International population reports. Washington, DC: U.S. Census Bureau; 2016.
3. Smith JS, Shaffrey CI, Berven S, et al. Operative versus nonoperative treatment of leg pain in adults with scoliosis: a retrospective review of a prospective multicenter database with two-year follow-up. Spine (Phila Pa 1976) 2009;34:1693–8.
4. Smith JS, Shaffrey CI, Berven S, et al. Improvement of back pain with operative and nonoperative treatment in adults with scoliosis. Neurosurgery 2009; 65:86–93.

5. Yadla S, Maltenfort MG, Ratliff JK, et al. Adult scoliosis surgery outcomes: a systematic review. Neurosurg Focus 2010;28:E3.

6. Street J, Lenehan B, DiPaola C, et al. Morbidity and mortality of major adult spinal surgery. A prospective cohort analysis of 942 consecutive patients. Spine J 2012;12:22–34.

7. Mummaneni PV, Shaffrey CI, Lenke LG, et al. The minimally invasive spinal deformity surgery algorithm: a reproducible rational framework for decision making in minimally invasive spinal deformity surgery. Neurosurg Focus 2014;36:E6.

8. Deukmedjian AR, Ahmadian A, Bach K, et al. Minimally invasive lateral approach for adult degenerative scoliosis: lessons learned. Neurosurg Focus 2013;35:E4.

9. Phillips FM, Isaacs RE, Rodgers WB, et al. Adult degenerative scoliosis treated with XLIF: clinical and radiographical results of a prospective multicenter study with 24-month follow-up. Spine (Phila Pa 1976) 2013;38:1853–61.

10. Daubs MD, Lenke LG, Bridwell KH, et al. Does correction of preoperative coronal imbalance make a difference in outcomes of adult patients with deformity? Spine (Phila Pa 1976) 2013;38:476–83.

11. Glassman SD, Berven S, Bridwell K, et al. Correlation of radiographic parameters and clinical symptoms in adult scoliosis. Spine (Phila Pa 1976) 2005; 30:682–8.

12. Costanzo G, Zoccali C, Maykowski P, et al. The role of minimally invasive lateral lumbar interbody fusion in sagittal balance correction and spinal deformity. Eur Spine J 2014;23:699–704.

13. Wang MY, Mummaneni PV, Fu KM, et al, Minimally Invasive Surgery Section of the International Spine Study Group. Less invasive surgery for treating adult spinal deformities: ceiling effects for deformity correction with 3 different techniques. Neurosurg Focus 2014;36:E12.

14. Strom RG, Bae J, Mizutani J, et al. Lateral interbody fusion combined with open posterior surgery for adult spinal deformity. J Neurosurg Spine 2016;25: 697–705.

15. Theologis AA, Mundis GM Jr, Nguyen S, et al. Utility of multilevel lateral interbody fusion of the thoracolumbar coronal curve apex in adult deformity surgery in combination with open posterior instrumentation and L5-S1 interbody fusion: a case-matched evaluation of 32 patients. J Neurosurg Spine 2017;26:208–19.

16. Deukmedjian AR, Dakwar E, Ahmadian A, et al. Early outcomes of minimally invasive anterior longitudinal ligament release for correction of sagittal imbalance in patients with adult spinal deformity. ScientificWorldJournal 2012;2012:789698.

17. Akbarnia BA, Mundis GM Jr, Moazzaz P, et al. Anterior column realignment (ACR) for focal kyphotic spinal deformity using a lateral transpsoas approach and ALL release. J Spinal Disord Tech 2014;27: 29–39.

18. Mundis GM Jr, Turner JD, Kabirian N, et al. Anterior column realignment has similar results to pedicle subtraction osteotomy in treating adults with sagittal plane deformity. World Neurosurg 2017;105:249–56.

19. Schwab FJ, Blondel B, Bess S, et al. Radiographical spinopelvic parameters and disability in the setting of adult spinal deformity: a prospective multicenter analysis. Spine (Phila Pa 1976) 2013;38:E803–12.

20. Protopsaltis T, Schwab F, Bronsard N, et al. The T1 pelvic angle, a novel radiographic measure of global sagittal deformity, accounts for both spinal inclination and pelvic tilt and correlates with health-related quality of life. J Bone Joint Surg Am 2014; 96:1631–40.

21. Kim YC, Lenke LG, Lee SJ, et al. The cranial sagittal vertical axis (CrSVA) is a better radiographic measure to predict clinical outcomes in adult spinal deformity surgery than the C7 SVA: a monocentric study. Eur Spine J 2017;26:2167–75.

22. Lafage R, Schwab F, Challier V, et al. Defining spinopelvic alignment thresholds: should operative goals in adult spinal deformity surgery account for age? Spine (Phila Pa 1976) 2016;41:62–8.

23. Uribe JS, Smith DA, Dakwar E, et al. Lordosis restoration after anterior longitudinal ligament release and placement of lateral hyperlordotic interbody cages during the minimally invasive lateral transpsoas approach: a radiographic study in cadavers. J Neurosurg Spine 2012;17:476–85.

24. Turner JD, Akbarnia BA, Eastlack RK, et al. Radiographic outcomes of anterior column realignment for adult sagittal plane deformity: a multicenter analysis. Eur Spine J 2015;24:427–32.

25. Bao H, Yan P, Qiu Y, et al. Coronal imbalance in degenerative lumbar scoliosis: prevalence and influence on surgical decision-making for spine osteotomy. Bone Joint J 2016;98:1227–33.

26. Oliveira L, Marchi L, Coutinho E, et al. A radiographic assessment of the ability of the extreme lateral interbody fusion procedure to indirectly decompress the neural elements. Spine (Phila Pa 1976) 2010;35:331–7.

27. Isaacs RE, Sembrano JN, Tohmeh AG, et al. Two-year comparative outcomes of MIS lateral and MIS transforaminal interbody fusion in the treatment of degenerative spondylolisthesis: part II: radiographic findings. Spine (Phila Pa 1976) 2016;41:133–44.

28. Elowitz EH, Yanni DS, Chwajol M, et al. Evaluation of indirect decompression of the lumbar spinal canal following minimally invasive lateral transpsoas interbody fusion: radiographic and outcome analysis. Minim Invasive Neurosurg 2011;54:201–6.

29. Regev GJ, Chen L, Dhawan M, et al. Morphometric analysis of the ventral nerve roots and

retroperitoneal vessels with respect to the minimally invasive lateral approach in normal and deformed spines. Spine (Phila Pa 1976) 2009;34:1330–5.

30. Louie PK, Narain AS, Hijji FY, et al. Radiographic analysis of psoas morphology and its association with neurovascular structures at l4-5 with reference to lateral approaches. Spine (Phila Pa 1976) 2017; 42(24):E1386–92.

31. O'Brien J, Haines C, Dooley ZA, et al. Femoral nerve strain at L4-L5 is minimized by hip flexion and increased by table break when performing lateral interbody fusion. Spine (Phila Pa 1976) 2014;39:33–8.

32. Yen CP, Uribe JS. Procedural checklist for retroperitoneal transpsoas minimally invasive lateral interbody fusion. Spine (Phila Pa 1976) 2016;41:152–8.

33. Ozgur BM, Aryan HE, Pimenta L, et al. Extreme lateral interbody fusion (XLIF): a novel surgical technique for anterior lumbar interbody fusion. Spine J 2006;6:435–43.

34. Dakwar E, Vale FL, Uribe JS. Trajectory of the main sensory and motor branches of the lumbar plexus outside the psoas muscle related to the lateral retroperitoneal transpsoas approach. J Neurosurg Spine 2011;14:290–5.

35. Uribe JS, Arredondo N, Dakwar E, et al. Defining the safe working zones using the minimally invasive lateral retroperitoneal transpsoas approach: an anatomical study. J Neurosurg Spine 2010;13: 260–6.

36. Tohmeh AG, Rodgers WB, Peterson MD, et al. Dynamically evoked, discrete-threshold electromyography in the extreme lateral interbody fusion approach. J Neurosurg Spine 2011;14:31–7.

37. Berjano P, Lamartina C. Minimally invasive lateral transpsoas approach with advanced neurophysiologic monitoring for lumbar interbody fusion. Eur Spine J 2011;20:1584–6.

38. Calancie B, Madsen P, Lebwohl N. Stimulus-evoked EMG monitoring during transpedicular lumbosacral spine instrumentation. Initial clinical results. Spine (Phila Pa 1976) 1994;19:2780–6.

39. Maguire J, Wallace S, Madiga R, et al. Evaluation of intrapedicular screw position using intraoperative evoked electromyography. Spine (Phila Pa 1976) 1995;20:1068–74.

40. Uribe JS, Isaacs RE, Youssef JA, et al. Can triggered electromyography monitoring throughout retraction predict postoperative symptomatic neuropraxia after XLIF? Results from a prospective multicenter trial. Eur Spine J 2015;24:378–85.

41. Cummock MD, Vanni S, Levi AD, et al. An analysis of postoperative thigh symptoms after minimally invasive transpsoas lumbar interbody fusion. J Neurosurg Spine 2011;15:11–8.

42. Abel NA, Januszewski J, Vivas AC, et al. Femoral nerve and lumbar plexus injury after minimally invasive lateral retroperitoneal transpsoas approach: electrodiagnostic prognostic indicators and a roadmap to recovery. Neurosurg Rev 2018;41:457–64.

43. Lykissas MG, Aichmair A, Hughes AP, et al. Nerve injury after lateral lumbar interbody fusion: a review of 919 treated levels with identification of risk factors. Spine J 2014;14:749–58.

44. Dakwar E, Le TV, Baaj AA, et al. Abdominal wall paresis as a complication of minimally invasive lateral transpsoas interbody fusion. Neurosurg Focus 2011;31:E18.

45. Uribe JS, Deukmedjian AR. Visceral, vascular, and wound complications following over 13,000 lateral interbody fusions: a survey study and literature review. Eur Spine J 2015;24:386–96.

46. Le TV, Baaj AA, Dakwar E, et al. Subsidence of polyetheretherketone intervertebral cages in minimally invasive lateral retroperitoneal transpsoas lumbar interbody fusion. Spine (Phila Pa 1976) 2012;37: 1268–73.

Lateral Prepsoas (Oblique) Approach Nuances

Anthony M. DiGiorgio, DO, MHA[a],*, Caleb S. Edwards, BA[b], Michael S. Virk, MD, PhD[c], Dean Chou, MD[d]

KEYWORDS

- Lumbar fusion • Interbody fusion • Prepsoas • Lumbar spine

KEY POINTS

- The prepsoas oblique approach to the lumbar spine provides many of the same benefits as the transpsoas lateral approach. This approach may decrease some of the complications seen with traversing the psoas muscle, such as femoral nerve traction.
- The oblique angle of this approach does not allow for perpendicular access to the spine. This can be challenging for surgeon orientation and navigation may help to orient the surgeon.
- This approach typically cannot be performed from the right side due to the position of the vena cava.
- A high-riding iliac crest is not a contraindication to this approach.
- This approach is a valuable tool for the surgeon in treating lumbar degenerative disease, low-grade spondylolisthesis, and coronal scoliosis.

INTRODUCTION

Interbody fusion can be an important tool to address lumbar spine pathology. In patients undergoing lumbar fusion, the addition of an interbody graft is suggested by the American Association of Neurological Surgeons (AANS) and Congress of Neurological Surgeons (CNS) guidelines on lumbar fusion.[1] There are many surgical approaches to interbody grafting of the lumbar spine including anterior, posterior, and lateral. Each approach has unique advantages and disadvantages.

A lateral approach allows for insertion of an interbody graft that spans the apophyseal ring.

This approach also lends itself to significant correction of coronal deformity.

Traversing the psoas muscle, however, has been associated with complications, such as muscle trauma, and damage to the lumbar plexus, genitofemoral, iliohypogastric, or ilioinguinal nerves. These complications can lead to sensory or motor changes to the thigh and leg.[2–5] In some patients, these changes can be permanent and debilitating. In addition, access to the L4-5 level can be challenging, and occasionally impossible, if a patient has a high-riding iliac crest.

The prepsoas, retroperitoneal approach, first described by Mayer in 1997,[6] provides an

Disclosure Statement: Dr D. Chou is a consultant for Medtronic and Globus and has received royalties from Globus. Dr M.S. Virk is a consultant for Globus; Dr A.M. DiGiorgio and Mr C.S. Edwards have no disclosures.
[a] Department of Neurosurgery, Louisiana State University Health Sciences Center, 2020 Gravier Street, 7th Floor, New Orleans, LA 70120, USA; [b] Department of Neurological Surgery, School of Medicine, University of California, San Francisco, 505 Parnassus Avenue, Room 779 M, San Francisco, CA 94143, USA; [c] Department of Neurological Surgery, Weill Cornell Medicine, New York Presbyterian, 525 East 68th Street, Starr 651, Box 99, New York, NY 10065, USA; [d] Department of Neurological Surgery, University of California, San Francisco, 505 Parnassus Avenue, Box 0112, San Francisco, CA 94143, USA
* Corresponding author.
E-mail address: adigi2@lsuhsc.edu

alternate lateral approach without traversing the psoas. By accessing the spine anteriorly to the psoas, it offers many of the benefits of the transpsoas approach while eliminating some of the associated risks. The prepsoas approach, also known as the oblique lateral interbody fusion (OLIF), allows access to L5-S1 with the assistance of an approach surgeon. See **Fig. 1** for a depiction of the access corridor in the prepsoas approach.

The approach can be done using fluoroscopy or CT-guided navigation. One potential advantage of navigation allows the surgeon to correct for the unfamiliar oblique trajectory and to decrease radiation exposure to the operative team.[7–9]

INDICATIONS/CONTRAINDICATIONS
Indications

Patients who meet the indications for lumbar interbody fusion may be considered for the prepsoas approach. These include 1 to 2 levels of degenerative spondylolisthesis refractory to conservative

management. L5-S1 may also be considered for this approach with the assistance of a vascular surgeon given the risk of vascular injury is much greater at this level.

Patients with coronal plane scoliosis with stenosis are also candidates for this approach. The prepsoas approach allows for indirect foraminal decompression by increasing the disk space height.

Contraindications

Due to the location of the vena cava, the risk of vascular injury precludes a right-sided approach for this procedure. Thus, patients with a concave coronal deformity on the right are not suited for a right-sided prepsoas approach. Lack of an operative corridor (as assessed on preoperative imaging showing vascular or visceral structures impeding access) is also a contraindication for this procedure.[10] A space must exist between the psoas and the aorta at the level of interest.

See **Table 1** for a summary.

SURGICAL TECHNIQUE/PROCEDURE
Preoperative Planning

- MRI is used to evaluate disks, neural elements and soft tissue. The corridor between the vena cava/iliac veins and the disk space needs to be evaluated.
  - See **Table 2** for the average size of that corridor as measured in an anatomic study by Davis and colleagues.[10]
- CT can be used to evaluate bony anatomy or in patients who cannot undergo an MRI.
- Three-ft standing radiographs to evaluate spinopelvic alignment and the position of the iliac crest
- Flexion/extension radiographs to evaluate for abnormal movement

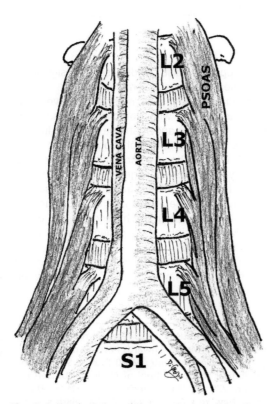

Fig. 1. Artist depiction of the prepsoas corridor. Note the position of the vena cava on the right side. This illustrates why the approach cannot be used from that side. The disk spaces are highlighted in yellow. (*Courtesy of* Anthony M. DiGiorgio, DO, MHA, New Orleans, LA.)

Table 1
Typical indications and contraindications of the prepsoas approach

Indications	Contraindications
1–2 levels of degenerative low-grade spondylolisthesis	Right-sided concave coronal deformity
Coronal plane scoliosis with stenosis	Lack of an operative corridor due to iliac vessel position seen on imaging

Table 2	
The average distances from the retracted psoas muscle to the aorta at each level during the prepsoas approach	
Level	**Mean Distance from Retracted Psoas to Vessel (mm)**
L2-3	25.5 ± 7.39
L3-4	27.1 ± 8.39
L4-5	24.5 ± 8.80

Data from Davis TT, Hynes RA, Fung DA, et al. Retroperitoneal oblique corridor to the L2-S1 intervertebral discs in the lateral position: an anatomic study. J Neurosurg Spine 2014;21(5):785–93.

Preparation and Patient Positioning

- The patient is induced under general anesthesia and intubated. Long-acting paralytics should not be used to avoid interference with intraoperative neuromonitoring.
- Neuromonitoring with free-running electromyography (EMG), motor-evoked potentials (MEPs), and somatosensory evoked potentials (SSEPs) are often used at the authors' institution
  - Although the risk of femoral nerve injury is low, EMG and MEP can alert the surgeon if the lumbar plexus is being compromised.
  - SSEP can be useful as an additional modality to address false-positive results.
- The patient is positioned in the right lateral decubitus position with the left side up (**Fig. 2**).
  - An axillary roll is placed along the chest wall, below the axilla, to protect the brachial plexus.
  - All pressure points are meticulously padded and the patient's trunk is stabilized by wrapping tape directly to the table. Care must be taken to not tape the legs too

tightly to avoid pressure, which could cause common peroneal nerve injury in the right leg.
  - A neutral position of the legs relaxes the psoas muscle and allows for easier retraction.
- The posterior superior iliac spine (PSIS) is marked and the patient is prepped and draped.

Surgical Approach

- The PSIS marking is identified and the reference array is placed approximately 5 cm superolateral to this point, along the iliac crest.
- Intraoperative CT is obtained and registered to navigation (**Fig. 3**).
- Intraoperative navigation is used to plan the incision. A virtual extension on the navigation probe is used to locate the midportion of the pathologic disk space. A true lateral from this is marked and a measurement is taken 5 cm anterior to this point (**Fig. 4**).
  - This marks the incision for the oblique approach. For L4-5, especially if the patient has a high iliac crest, this incision may be carried anteriorly an additional 2 cm.
- The incision is made obliquely, parallel to the trajectories of the abdominal wall nerve roots. This is carried down to the abdominal fascia in a trajectory toward the lumbar spine.
  - Navigation can be routinely used to verify trajectory and position.
- Handheld retractors are used to visualize dissection through the external oblique, internal oblique and transversus abdominus.
  - Blunt dissection is used rather than electrocautery to protect the nerves in the abdominal wall. This can safely be done using hemostats or scissors.

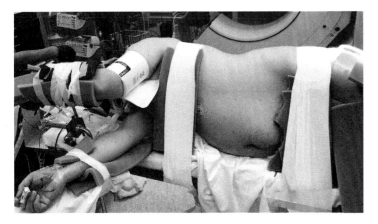

Fig. 2. The patient is positioned in the lateral decubitus position with the left side up and securely taped to the bed. All pressure points are meticulously padded.

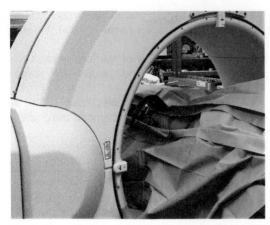

Fig. 3. The reference array has been placed in the PSIS and the intraoperative CT scanner has entered the field to obtain images.

- The retroperitoneal fat is seen deep to the transverses abdominis muscles. Finger dissection is used to sweep the retroperitoneal fat and peritoneal contents off the posterior abdominal wall and over the psoas muscle (**Fig. 5**). Navigation is used to verify the correct level as well as to identify the anterior border of the psoas.
- The psoas can be gently mobilized posteriorly.
- The disk space is cleared of soft tissue using blunt instruments.
- Sequential dilators are placed and triggered EMG is used to confirm adequate distance from the lumbar plexus. A table mounted retractor is then inserted and locked into place.
- Annulotomy and discectomy are performed.
  ○ A straight trajectory from this oblique angle can injure the contralateral nerve root, and, thus, as the instruments are placed into the disk space at an oblique angle, they are rotated posteriorly until they pass in the true lateral position, despite the oblique approach.
    ▪ The surgeon must move the hand dorsally to correct for the oblique angle (**Figs. 6** and **7**).

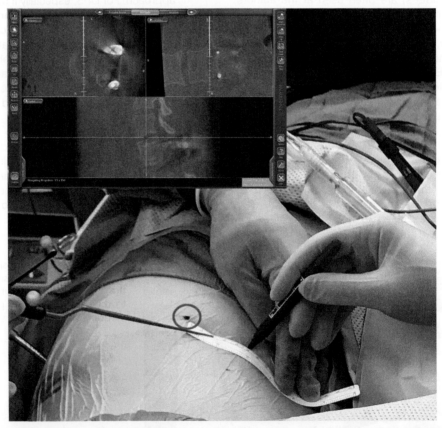

Fig. 4. The incision is planned by marking the operative disk space in a true lateral position using navigation. That mark is highlighted here with the red circle and the location on navigation is seen in the inset. The incision is drawn 5 cm anterior to that.

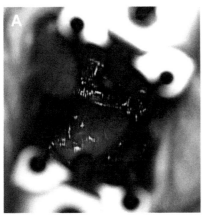 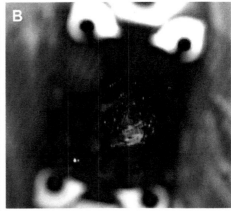

Fig. 5. A view of the dissection through the prepsoas corridor. Retroperitoneal fat is seen in (*A*). This is swept off, revealing the fascia overlying the lumbar spine. Once cleared, the disk space can be seen (*B*).

- Thorough discectomy is performed and end plates are prepared. A Cobb elevator is used to break through the contralateral annulus.

- Navigated interbody template trials are placed.
- The correctly sized implant is loaded with graft material and placed with navigation as well. This confirms correct trajectory and placement spanning the apophyseal ring.
- Fluoroscopy is used to verify interbody position if navigation shifted during the operation.
- The retractor is slowly removed and the wound is closed in a layered fashion.

COMPLICATIONS AND MANAGEMENT

Complications with the prepsoas approach are similar to those from both the ALIF and transpsoas lateral approaches. If the peritoneum is violated, it should be repaired with a suture. Although the psoas is not traversed, working around it can still lead to paresis (from traction on the anterior margin when rotating instruments) or a psoas hematoma. Groin numbness and paresthesias have also been reported. Ileus, major vascular injury, sympathetic chain injury, and incisional hernia can all occur as well.[11] A painful, swollen leg postoperatively may indicate a sympathetic chain or vascular injury. Neurologic injury is always possible and postoperative imaging should be obtained if this is the case. A misplaced cage can impinge on the nerve root and requires reoperation and correction. Pseudarthrosis is a late complication that would also require reoperation.

Although L5-S1 can be accessed through the lateral, prepsoas approach, the rate of vascular injury increases at this level. An adequate corridor was only found in 70% of the MRI images analyzed by Molinares and colleagues.[12]

Fig. 6. Artist depiction of the orthogonal move to take instrumentation from an oblique approach to a lateral one. (*Courtesy of* Anthony M. DiGiorgio, DO, MHA, New Orleans, LA.)

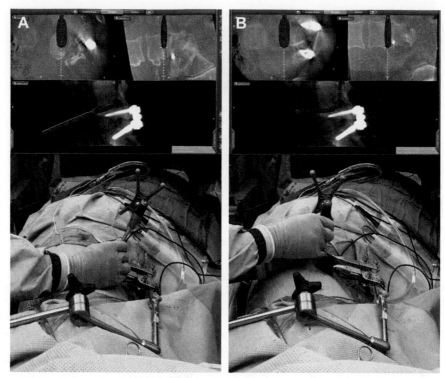

Fig. 7. The orthogonal move to bring instruments into a true lateral is seen here. (*A*) The photograph shows the disk space trial at an oblique angle and the superimposed navigation screen (*top panels*) depicts this. After moving the hand dorsally (*B*), the instrument has a more lateral trajectory, as confirmed with navigation (*top panels*).

Vascular injury to the aorta, iliac vessels, or segmental vessels may rarely occur and require conversion to open surgery for vascular repair.

Rarely, the ureter may be injured resulting in urinoma.

POSTOPERATIVE CARE

- Posterior instrumentation may be placed during the same procedure or staged. The authors typically use posterior pedicle screw fixation in all cases to reduce pseudarthrosis and subsidence.

Table 3
The demographics of 49 consecutive patients undergoing the prepsoas approach using navigation at University of California, San Francisco

Parameter	Number
Age range	31–89
Average age	66.8 ± 9.6
Female	31 (63.3%)
Total levels fused	
1	26 (53.1%)
2	13 (26.5%)
3	8 (16.3%)
4	2 (4.1%)
Posterior approach	
None	7 (14.3%)
Minimally invasive	18 (36.7%)
Open	24 (49.0%)
Staged posterior instrumentation	16 (32.7%)

Table 4
The surgical results from 49 patients undergoing the prepsoas approach using navigation at University of California, San Francisco

Parameter	Value
Complications	
Psoas hematoma	1
Transient thigh sensory changes	3
Ileus	3
Surgery time (min)	303 ± 159
Estimated blood loss (mL)	228 ± 225
Length of stay (days)	6 ± 3

Table 5
Preoperative and postoperative back pain and leg pain as measured on the visual analog scale.

Value	Preoperative	Postoperative	P Value
VAS back pain	8.03 ± 2.11	3.41 ± 3.24	<.001
VAS leg pain	6.81 ± 3.29	1.44 ± 3.08	<.001

- ○ Staging the procedure allows for clinical assessment of the efficacy of indirect decompression if radiculopathy has improved.
- Postoperatively, the patients are mobilized on day 1. A clear liquid diet is given until bowel movement, at which time regular diet is given. Patients are discharged home once they are adequately mobilizing, having bowel movements, and pain is controlled with oral medication.

OUTCOMES

For results from 49 consecutive patients undergoing the navigated pre-psoas approach at the University of California, San Francisco, See **Tables 3–5**. Average follow up was one year in this series.

SUMMARY

Approaching the lumbar spine anterior to the psoas, or obliquely, decreases the risk of damaging the psoas muscle and the nerves that run within it. Along with the lumbar plexus, sensory nerves (which traverse outside the psoas and directly in the path of a transpsoas approach) innervating the thigh are also at risk with the transpsoas approach.[13,14] The lumbar plexus can be somewhat protected with triggered EMG and MEP monitoring, both with the prepsoas and transpsoas approaches. The small cutaneous nerves, however, do not have a motor component and thus cannot be detected with neuromonitoring. The rate of sensory deficits is reported to be as high as 27.1% when traversing the psoas.[15] Although this risk is not completely avoided with the prepsoas approach, it is decreased to approximately 6%.[7] This is why it is important to use blunt dissection after entering the fascia of the abdominal wall. Electrocautery should not be used past this point.

The angle for the prepsoas approach can also be unfamiliar to the surgeon. With anterior, posterior, or lateral transpsoas approaches, the surgeon operates at a true perpendicular angle to the spine. Operating at an oblique angle can make orientation of vital structures more difficult. Navigation allows the surgeon to identify vital structures and ensure proper trajectory. This is one advantage of navigation for this approach, in addition to reducing radiation exposure to the patient and operative team.

The prepsoas approach also allows for access to L5-S1 from the lateral position. A trained approach surgeon is used because of the proximity of the left iliac vein. Preoperative imaging needs to be assessed for the operative corridor as well as for the morphology of the sacral slope and iliac crest. Not all patients have an adequate corridor and some may have bony morphology that prohibits an adequate operative angle.

Posterior fixation can be performed if indicated. This can be done open or minimally invasive and staged if needed. Staging the posterior portion allows assessment of any residual radicular pain after indirect decompression. If the patient still has radiculopathy, open posterior fixation allows for direct decompression at the same time the instrumentation is placed.

This approach is a valuable tool for surgeons in treating lumbar degenerative disease or coronal scoliosis with stenosis. It is not meant to replace the anterior, posterior, or transpsoas approaches but rather provides another option in tailoring of the optimal treatment of each patient.

REFERENCES

1. Mummaneni PV, Dhall SS, Eck JC, et al. Guideline update for the performance of fusion procedures for degenerative disease of the lumbar spine. Part 11: interbody techniques for lumbar fusion. J Neurosurg Spine 2014;21(1):67–74.
2. Moller DJ, Slimack NP, Acosta FL Jr, et al. Minimally invasive lateral lumbar interbody fusion and transpsoas approach-related morbidity. Neurosurg Focus 2011;31(4):E4.
3. Ozgur BM, Aryan HE, Pimenta L, et al. Extreme lateral interbody fusion (XLIF): a novel surgical technique for anterior lumbar interbody fusion. Spine J 2006;6(4):435–43.
4. Rodgers WB, Gerber EJ, Patterson J. Intraoperative and early postoperative complications in extreme lateral interbody fusion: an analysis of 600 cases. Spine 2011;36(1):26–32.
5. Ohtori S, Orita S, Yamauchi K, et al. Mini-open anterior retroperitoneal lumbar interbody fusion: oblique lateral interbody fusion for lumbar spinal degeneration disease. Yonsei Med J 2015;56(4):1051–9.
6. Mayer HM. A new microsurgical technique for minimally invasive anterior lumbar interbody fusion. Spine 1997;22(6):691–9 [discussion: 700].

7. DiGiorgio AM, Edwards CS, Virk MS, et al. Stereotactic navigation for the prepsoas oblique lateral lumbar interbody fusion: technical note and case series. Neurosurg focus 2017;43(2):E14.

8. Villard J, Ryang YM, Demetriades AK, et al. Radiation exposure to the surgeon and the patient during posterior lumbar spinal instrumentation: a prospective randomized comparison of navigated versus non-navigated freehand techniques. Spine 2014; 39(13):1004–9.

9. Zhang YH, White I, Potts E, et al. Comparison perioperative factors during minimally invasive prepsoas lateral interbody fusion of the lumbar spine using either navigation or conventional fluoroscopy. Glob Spine J 2017;7(7):657–63.

10. Davis TT, Hynes RA, Fung DA, et al. Retroperitoneal oblique corridor to the L2-S1 intervertebral discs in the lateral position: an anatomic study. J Neurosurg Spine 2014;21(5):785–93.

11. Silvestre C, Mac-Thiong J-M, Hilmi R, et al. Complications and morbidities of mini-open anterior retroperitoneal lumbar interbody fusion: oblique lumbar interbody fusion in 179 patients. Asian Spine J 2012;6(2):89–97.

12. Molinares DM, Davis TT, Fung DA. Retroperitoneal oblique corridor to the L2-S1 intervertebral discs: an MRI study. J Neurosurg Spine 2016;24(2): 248–55.

13. Mobbs RJ, Phan K, Malham G, et al. Lumbar interbody fusion: techniques, indications and comparison of interbody fusion options including PLIF, TLIF, MI-TLIF, OLIF/ATP, LLIF and ALIF. J Spine Surg (Hong Kong) 2015;1(1):2–18.

14. Cummock MD, Vanni S, Levi AD, et al. An analysis of postoperative thigh symptoms after minimally invasive transpsoas lumbar interbody fusion. J Neurosurg Spine 2011;15(1):11–8.

15. Joseph JR, Smith BW, La Marca F, et al. Comparison of complication rates of minimally invasive transforaminal lumbar interbody fusion and lateral lumbar interbody fusion: a systematic review of the literature. Neurosurg focus 2015;39(4):E4.

Anterior Column Release/Realignment

David S. Xu, MD[a], Jason Paluzzi, MD[b], Adam S. Kanter, MD[c], Juan S. Uribe, MD[a,d],*

KEYWORDS

- Osteotomy • Spine deformity • MIS • Spine surgery • Scoliosis • XLIF

KEY POINTS

- Anterior column release/realignment (ACR) is a powerful tool to increase lumbar lordosis by lengthening the anterior column.
- Minimally invasive lateral ACR can achieve large corrections at a single segment.
- Posterior column facet osteotomies combined with lateral ACR increase segmental lordosis and can match the corrections achieved with a conventional 3-column osteotomy.
- Lumbar lordosis and other radiographic outcomes after lateral ACR are durable up to 20 months after surgery based on the authors' experience.

INTRODUCTION

Restoration of sagittal balance and spinopelvic harmony is vital in the management of adult spinal deformity. As patients lose lumbar lordosis (LL) through disk degeneration and vertebral body insufficiency, they are forced to maintain their center of balance by compensatory mechanisms, such as thoracic hypokyphosis and pelvic retroversion.[1–4] Failure of these mechanisms results in progressive mismatch between a patient's LL and pelvic incidence (PI), ultimately leading to increasing positive sagittal vertical axis (SVA). This inability to maintain posture with the head over the pelvis results in debilitating pain, impaired mobility, loss of a level forward gaze, and overall reduced function and quality of life. When addressed surgically, spinal alignment for most adults should be corrected to have an SVA of less than or equal to 5 cm, pelvic tilt (PT) less than 25°, and an LL within 10° of the PI.[2,5,6]

Traditionally, multiple posterior osteotomy techniques have been used to restore segmental lordosis to the spine by destabilizing and shortening the posterior spinal column.[7] Within the past decade, however, greater attention has turned toward surgical strategies aimed at lengthening the anterior column through release of the anterior longitudinal ligament (ALL) and placement of a large, hyperlordotic interbody. The prototypical technique is an extension of the minimally invasive surgery (MIS) lateral lumbar interbody fusion (LLIF), where the ALL can be safely dissected and released from a lateral approach, but other anterior and posterior approaches have also emerged. As a collective, these surgical strategies are referred to as anterior column release/realignment (ACR).

Beginning with adoption of the lateral ACR technique through the transpsoas LLIF approach, access to the anterior lumbar spine with overall reduced operative time and morbidity has become

Disclosures: Dr J.S. Uribe is a consultant for NuVasive.
Financial Support: None.
[a] Department of Neurological Surgery, Barrow Neurological Institute, St. Joseph's Hospital and Medical Center, 350 West Thomas Road, Phoenix, AZ 85013, USA; [b] Department of Neurosurgery and Brain Repair, University of South Florida, 2 Tampa General Circle, Tampa, FL 33606, USA; [c] Department of Neurological Surgery, University of Pittsburgh Medical Center, 200 Lothrop Street, Pittsburgh, PA 15212, USA; [d] Division of Spinal Disorders, St. Joseph's Hospital and Medical Center, 350 West Thomas Road, Phoenix, AZ 85013, USA
* Corresponding author. Division of Spinal Disorders, St. Joseph's Hospital and Medical Center, 350 West Thomas Road, Phoenix, AZ 85013.
E-mail address: juansuribe@gmail.com

Neurosurg Clin N Am 29 (2018) 427–437
https://doi.org/10.1016/j.nec.2018.03.008
1042-3680/18/© 2018 Elsevier Inc. All rights reserved.

more feasible with powerful correction of global spinal alignment on par with traditional posterior osteotomies.[8–13] Early outcomes of MIS lateral ACR demonstrated a 10° to 27° increase in segmental lordosis and 16° to 31° increase in mean global lordosis, with complication rates varying from 18% to 48%, with a 5.3% risk of proximal junctional kyphosis (PJK).[14] Long-term results regarding surgical outcome of MIS ACR remain lacking. Within this review, the authors present an overview of the current lateral ACR technique from surgical planning to execution and evaluate long-term radiographic outcomes from their personal case series.

PATIENT SELECTION

A summary of indications and contraindications for ACR is included in **Table 1**. A lateral ACR provides indirect decompression of the thecal sac, neuroforamen, and restores significant segmental lordosis greater than what is typically achievable through a standard LLIF. Consequently, the predominant indication for performing an ACR rather than a traditional LLIF is to provide segmental lordosis exceeding 10° for correction of spinal deformities. Specifically, previous work reported by Mummaneni and colleagues[15] delineated a framework for determining the deformity patient population that is most amenable for an MIS treatment strategy. Patients ideally should have an SVA less than 6 cm unless their curve is flexible, PT less than 25°, PI-LL mismatch between 10° and 30°, maximum coronal Cobb angle less than 20°, and thoracic kyphosis less than 60°.[15] Treatment of patients outside of these parameters is possible but should be reviewed by multiple surgeons and attempted only by experienced providers.

In principle, the T12-L5 segments can be accessed laterally for an ACR, but in practice a majority of ACRs are performed at L2-5 to reapproximate the distribution of segmental lordosis in the lumbar spine. Contraindications for a lateral ACR

include extensive previous surgeries involving retroperitoneal structures, such as the kidneys and ascending/descending colon. Because interbody subsidence is a prominent source of treatment failure, a lateral ACR should be avoided in patients with severe osteopenia or osteoporosis. The authors prefer patients to be evaluated with dual-energy x-ray absorptiometry (DEXA) and have femoral neck T-scores greater than −2.0. Lastly, caution and close evaluation of preoperative imaging must be performed when planning to intervene at L4-5 in patients with transitional anatomy due to anterior displacement of the lumbar plexus.

TECHNIQUE

A lateral ACR uses much of the same workflow as a transpsoas LLIF but with greater risk to the great vessels and peritoneal structures. Therefore, surgeons attempting an ACR should first be adept and comfortable with the classic retroperitoneal, transpsoas LLIF approach. First described by Pimenta and colleagues,[16] the LLIF initially entailed a transpsoas dissection through endoscope assisted direct visualization but has since evolved into multiple minimally invasive platforms, such as the Extreme Lateral Interbody Fusion (XLIF) (NuVasive, San Diego, California) and Direct Lateral Interbody Fusion (DLIF) (Medtronic, Memphis, Tennessee). These contemporary systems rely on fluoroscopically assisted passage of a blunt dissector through the psoas muscle that is sequentially dilated to expose the lateral aspect of the disk space. Directional electromyographic (EMG) neuromonitoring further allows active neuromonitoring to ensure that the dilators and retractor are anterior to the lumbar plexus, aiding in prevention of retraction related injury.

Preoperative Evaluation

Prior to surgery, close scrutiny of MRI and CT imaging should be performed to determine the optimal side of approach and relationship of

Table 1
Indications and contraindications of lateral anterior column release

Indications	Contraindications

• Location: T12-L5 disk spaces
• Need for segmental lordosis >10°
• Radiographic parameters:
  ○ SVA <6 cm unless the curve is flexible
  ○ PT <25°
  ○ PI-LL mismatch 10°30°
  ○ Cobb angle <20°
  ○ Thoracic kyphosis <60°
	• Fused or previously instrumented disk space
	• Transitional anatomy at L4-5
	• T-score >2.0 measured at the femoral neck
	• Previous retroperitoneal surgery
	• No tissue plane between vertebral body and ventral vessels assessed on preoperative imaging

vascular structures to the spine. It is important to account for all vessels in line with the plane of dissection, even those across the disk space to avoid injury when performing the contralateral annulotomy (**Fig. 1**A). Attention should also be given to the ventral vessels to assess whether an adventitial plane of dissection exists between the vessels and the disk space.

Patient Positioning

Patients are positioned in the lateral decubitus position with the iliac crest at the level of the table break and the side of approach facing upwards. The hips and knees are flexed to relax the psoas muscle, and rolls are positioned under the axilla to decompress the brachia plexus and just above the down-facing iliac crest to facilitate flexion of the torso (**Fig. 1**B). Fluoroscopy is brought in to aid in patient and table positioning so that perfect anterior-posterior and lateral radiographs can be obtained without adjustment of the fluoroscopy machine's rotational or tilt angles. A transverse incision is planned to overlie the lateral projection of the disk space on the patient's flank, centered on 50% of the anterior-posterior endplate length.

Lateral Approach and Diskectomy

At the start of surgery, the incision is opened, and electrocautery is used to expose and divide the facia of the external oblique. Access to the retroperitoneum is gained by blunt dissection through the lateral muscle layers with 2 tonsil hemostats, followed by gentle puncture through the transversalis fascia. Finger dissection is then used to develop the retroperitoneal space by sweeping the peritoneal structures anteriorly and to guide the initial dilators to the superficial surface of the psoas muscle. Fluoroscopy and EMG neuromonitoring facilitate passage of the initial dilator to overlie the lateral surface of the disk space at the 50% anterior-posterior length and anterior to the lumbar plexus (**Fig. 2**A). Sequential dilation is performed, and the lateral access retractor is placed with fluoroscopic and radiographic verification of its positioning (**Fig. 2**B). On successful access to the lateral disk space, a generous annulotomy is made just posterior to the ALL, and diskectomy is performed, followed by a contralateral annulotomy with a cobb elevator and, finally, curettage of the cartilaginous endplates to facilitate arthrodesis (**Fig. 2**C).

Anterior Phase

After diskectomy, a blunt dissector, such as Penfield #4 or Endoscopic Kittner, is used to dissect the adventitial plane ventral to the disk space and ALL. Development of this plane is critical to protect the ventral vasculature. The dissection should proceed to a depth equal to the contralateral pedicle and can be verified with fluoroscopy. After this surgical plane has been created, an anterior retractor is inserted along its length and a long-handle blade or disk cutter is then slowly advanced behind the retractor to cut the ALL (**Fig. 3**A). Anterior-posterior fluoroscopy is vital to ensure that the blade does not traverse farther than the length of the anterior dissector. Typically, only 75% of the ALL length needs to be cut. After incision of the ALL, a disk space spreader or sequentially larger trials are inserted into the disk space to distract the vertebral body and propagate the ALL incision, leading to its full release

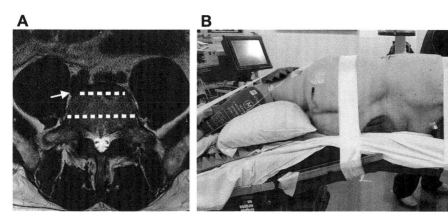

A   **B**

Fig. 1. Overview of lateral ACR. (*A*) An axial T2-weighted MRI slice of the L4-5 interspace shows an overview of the planned lateral trajectory of the diskectomy and interbody placement (*grid lines*). A prevertebral vein is present within the working trajectory (*arrow*) and is at risk of injury with a left sided approach during the contralateral annulotomy. A right-sided approach allows visualization and control of the vessel during all parts of the procedure. (*B*) A lateral photo of a patient positioned for an LLIF. (*Courtesy of* Barrow Neurological Institute, Phoenix, AZ.)

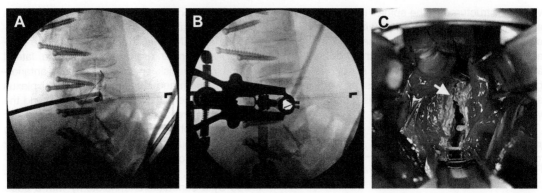

Fig. 2. Lateral ACR initial phase. (*A*) After gaining retroperitoneal access, a blunt dilator is passed through the psoas to rest on the lateral surface of the disk space at the 50% anterior-posterior length of the disk space. Some retractor systems allow directional triggered EMG monitoring to verify positioning of the dilator anterior to the lumbar plexus. (*B*) Sequential dilation is performed, and the lateral access retractor is passed through the transpsoas corridor to rest on the 50% anterior-posterior disk length. (*C*) On successful access to the lateral disk space, a generous annulotomy and diskectomy are performed is made just posterior to the ALL (*arrow*). (*Courtesy of* Barrow Neurological Institute, Phoenix, AZ.)

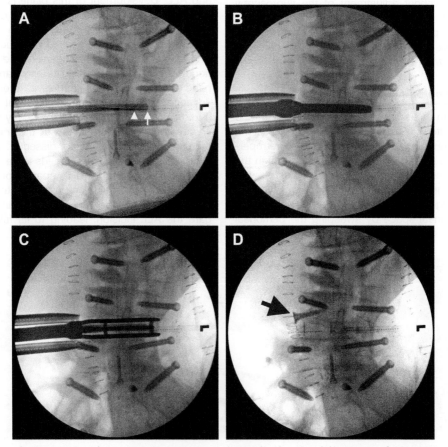

Fig. 3. Lateral ACR anterior phase. Anterior-posterior radiographs showing (*A*) passage of an anterior retractor blade (*arrow*) ventral to the disk space to protect the great vessels during resection of the ALL with a scalpel (*arrowhead*). After the ALL is cut, a disk space spreader is inserted into the diskectomy cavity (*B*) and expanded (*C*) to propagate the ALL incision until it is fully torn. A hyperlordoic interbody is inserted into the disk space with an integrated screw (*D*) A hyperlordoic interbody is inserted into the disk space with an integrated screw (*arrow*) applied to secure the implant and prevent it from migrating ventrally. (*Courtesy of* Barrow Neurological Institute, Phoenix, AZ.)

(Fig. 3B, C). An appropriately sized lordotic interbody is then inserted into the disk space. To prevent migration of the interbody ventrally, the authors recommend utilization of an implant that features in situ fixation, such as an integrated screw (Fig. 3D). After placement of the implant, the retractor is withdrawn under direct visualization to verify appropriate hemostasis and the incisions are closed. Posterior fixation with pedicle screws are then placed.

CASE EXAMPLE

A 70-year-old woman with debilitating back pain was evaluated in clinic. Her standing scoliosis radiographs (Figs. 4A, B) revealed a positive SVA of 15 cm, a PI of 44°, an LL of 4°, a PI-LL mismatch of 40°, a PT of 32°, and a maximal coronal Cobb angle of 52° measured from the superior endplate of L5 to the superior endplate of L1. The patient had a DEXA scan showing a femoral neck t-score of −2.6 and was not recommended surgery until after 6 months of teriparatide therapy, when a repeat DEXA scan showed a femoral neck t-score of −1.8.

A 2-stage, minimally invasive deformity correction surgery was planned. During stage 1, the patient underwent an L5-S1 anterior ACR, followed by percutaneous pedicle screw placement from T10 to ilium. During stage 2, the patient underwent a 2-level lateral ACR from L3-5, followed by an LLIF at L2-3 with rod fixation of the posterior pedicle screws (Fig. 4C, D). The anterior ACR provided 24° of segmental lordosis, and the 2-level lateral ACR provided an additional 22° of segmental lordosis. On her final postoperative standing scoliosis radiographs (Fig. 4E, F), the patient's SVA of 5 cm, a PI of 44°, an LL of 34°, a PI-LL mismatch of 10°, a PT of 17°, and a maximal coronal Cobb angle of 28°. The patient was discharged to acute in-patient rehabilitation and was released home after 9 weeks of therapy. At her discharge, the patient has no neurologic deficits and greatly improved ambulation and pain compared with before surgery.

MATERIALS AND METHODS
Patient Population

A retrospective review of all consecutive cases performed by the senior author (J.S.U.) from 2010 to 2015 was conducted to identify patients with adult degenerative spinal deformity who underwent surgical treatment involving a lateral ACR through an MIS retroperitoneal transpsoas approach at a single institution. Inclusion criteria included global spinal malalignment with an SVA greater than 5 cm or PI-LL mismatch greater than 10°, clinical and radiographic follow-up of at least 1-year in length, and a primary pathology of adult degenerative deformity. All patients underwent preoperative and postoperative standing anterior-posterior and lateral scoliosis radiographs as well as repeat imaging at each stage of follow-up at 6 weeks, 3 months, 6 months, and 12 months and annually thereafter.

Patient demographics and clinical outcomes were recorded. Parameters, including PI, LL, SVA, and PT, were measured preoperatively and at the most recent follow-up. Other characteristics analyzed included the presence of cage

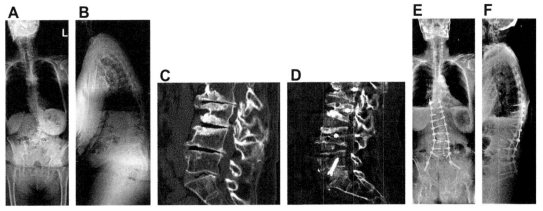

Fig. 4. Case example. Anterior-posterior (A) and lateral projection (B) scoliosis radiographs of a 70-year-old woman demonstrate a positive SVA of 15 cm, a PI of 44°, an LL of 4°, a PI-LL mismatch of 40°, a PT of 32°, and a maximal coronal Cobb angle of 52° from the superior endplate of L5 to the superior endplate of L1. Lateral slices of a lumbar spine CT scan (C) before and (D) after surgery demonstrate 24° of segmental lordosis achieved with an anterior ACR and an additional 22° of segmental lordosis achieved with a 2-level L3-5 lateral ACR. Anterior-posterior (E) and lateral projection (F) scoliosis radiographs obtained 1 week after surgery demonstrate an SVA of 5 cm, a PI of 44°, an LL of 34°, a PI-LL mismatch of 10°, a PT of 17°, and a maximal coronal Cobb angle of 28°. (Courtesy of Barrow Neurological Institute, Phoenix, AZ.)

subsidence, PJK, and evidence of arthrodesis. Preoperative and postoperative segmental lordosis and the use of a posterior osteotomy at the level of the ALL release were also recorded. The paired *t* test and Wilcoxon signed ranks test was used to analyze changes in continuous and ordinal clinical variables respectively. Statistically significant changes were defined as *P* values less than .05.

Proximal Junction Kyphosis Definition

The definition of PJK varies widely in the literature[17] with relation to the proximal junctional angle (PJA), defined as the sagittal Cobb angle of the inferior endplate of the upper instrumented vertebra to the superior endplate of the vertebra 2 levels above the upper instrumented vertebra. Studies examining PJK have variable thresholds for the PJA that range from 10° to 20°. To compare this study's data with the widest breadth of definitions available, the authors set a threshold for PJK at 2 different PJA thresholds: 5° and 20° changes from preoperative measurements. Proximal junctional failure (PJF) was defined as PJK requiring surgical revision.

RESULTS
Patient Characteristics and Follow-up

From 2010 to 2015, 73 adult spinal deformity patients underwent an MIS lateral ACR. Of these, 41 patients met the inclusion criteria for the study, with a total of 55 levels of ACR performed. Four (7.3%) ACRs were performed at the L1-2 level, 11 (20.0%) at L2-3, 27 (49.1%) at L3-4, and 13 (23.6%) at L4-5. The average patient age was 64.0 years, with a gender distribution of 56% female and 44% male. All patients underwent placement of a 30° hyperlordotic cage at the ACR level and supplemental posterior spinal fixation with pedicle

screws and rods. In addition, 21 (51.2%) patients underwent a posterior column osteotomy (PCO) composed of a complete inferior facetectomy at 29 (52.7%) ACR levels prior to placement of the lateral interbody to facilitate lordosis. The average duration of follow-up was 20 months (range 12–49 months).

Global Radiographic Outcomes

A summary of global radiographic changes is summarized in **Table 2**. At their last follow-up, all 41 patients maintained an increased global LL by an average of 16.7° (*P*<.001), a reduction in their baseline SVA by an average of 2.5 cm (*P* = .009), and a reduction in the PI-LL mismatch by an average of 15.1° (*P*<.001). Thoracic kyphosis corrected by an average of 7.3°. Fifteen patients (37%) demonstrated radiographic PJK with a PJA threshold of 5°, and 4 patients (9.8%) demonstrated radiographic PJK with a PJA threshold of 20°. A total of 4 (9.8%) patients in this cohort developed PJF, 3 from the less stringent PJK classification group and 1 from the more stringent classification group.

When dichotomizing the patient cohort into those who underwent a posterior osteotomy at the level of ACR versus those who did not, there was a statistically significant greater correction regarding the SVA (4.3 cm vs 0.6 cm), PI-LL mismatch (21.5° vs 8.3°), PT (8.1°vs 1.9°), and LL (23.5° vs 4.6°). Furthermore, a statistically significant higher incidence of interbody subsidence was seen among patients who underwent a posterior osteotomy versus those who did not (28.5% vs 10.0%).

Segmental Radiographic Outcomes

Table 3 outlines changes in segmental radiographic findings across the 55 ACR levels treated at the patients' last follow-up. The average

Table 2
Global radiographic outcomes

	All Patients (n = 41)	Without Posterior Column Osteotomy (n = 20)	With Posterior Column Osteotomy (n = 21)	P Value
Δ SVA (cm)	2.5	0.6	4.3	**.008**
Δ PI-LL (°)	15.1	8.3	21.5	**.004**
Δ PT (°)	5.16	1.9	8.1	**.02**
Δ LL (°)	16.7	9.6	23.5	**.002**
Δ TK (°)	7.3	4.6	9.9	.11
Subsidence (%)	8 (19.5)	2 (10.0)	6 (28.5)	**.02**
PJK (%, ΔPJA >5°)	15 (36.6)	6 (30.0)	9 (42.8)	.41
PJK (%, ΔPJA >20°)	4 (9.8)	1 (5.0)	3 (14.3)	.33
PJF (%)	4 (9.8)	1 (5.0)	3 (14.3)	.33

Abbreviation: TK, thoracic kyphosis. Bold formatting in the rightmost column signifies statistically significance (*P*<.05).

Table 3
Segmental radiographic outcomes

	Number of Patients			Δ Segmental Lordosis (°)				Subsidence n (%)			
	All	Levels Without Posterior Column Osteotomy	Levels with Posterior Column Osteotomy	All	Levels Without Posterior Column Osteotomy	Levels with Posterior Column Osteotomy	P Value	All	Levels Without Posterior Column Osteotomy	Levels with Posterior Column Osteotomy	P Value
L1/2	4	1	3	27.6	19.5	30.3	.013	1	0	1 (33.3)	<.001
L2/3	11	6	5	14.1	12.6	15.9		3	1 (16.7)	2 (40.0)	
L3/4	27	15	12	13.5	11.3	16.4		5	0	5 (41.6)	
L4/5	13	4	9	13.6	10.4	15.1		0	0	0	
All levels	55	26	29	14.7	11.8	17.3		9	1 (3.8)	8 (27.6)	

increase in segmental lordosis across the ACR level was 14.7°, with L1-2 demonstrating the highest average increase in segmental lordosis after ACR, with a gain of 27.6°. Patients undergoing a PCO at the ACR level demonstrated greater segmental lordosis gains at every treated level as well as an average statistically significant average increase of 5.5° (17.3° vs 11.8°; $P = .013$) across all levels. A total of 9 (16.4%) interbodies showed evidence of subsidence. Most subsided cages (8 of 9) occurred at treated levels that had previously undergone a posterior osteotomy.

At 1-year postprocedure, plain radiographs to evaluate fusion was available for 52 (92.5%) treated levels. Based on the Bridwell classification, where grade I and II findings indicate fusion, 49 of the 52 levels (94.2%) showed radiographic evidence of arthrodesis.

Adverse Events

No patients experienced serious vascular or visceral complications from the ACR procedure. Similarly, no patients experienced permanent neurologic, strength, or sensory deficits. One patient experienced transient thigh numbness that resolved within the first month after surgery.

DISCUSSION
Lordosis Gains with Anterior Column Release

Traditionally, extensive multicolumn osteotomies were used to restore LL in adult spinal deformity. Recently, Schwab and colleagues[7] organized posterior osteotomies into a comprehensive classification system in progressive order of complexity, destabilization, and gains in segmental lordosis. Within that classification system, 3-column osteotomies, encompassing pedicle subtraction and corpectomies, provide the greatest amount of LL, often exceeding 25° per level, but are very morbid.[18] A recent historical review of 573 patients underwent a 3-column osteotomy revealed that within the most recent time period of 2010 to 2013, major complications had an incidence of 39% and blood loss exceeding 4 L occurred 16.7% of the time.[19]

From the authors' patient cohort and within a growing body of literature, lateral ACR has demonstrated the ability to restore significant lordosis at approxiamtely 10° per level without posterior osteotomies.[20] When combined with posterior osteotomies, which can be done in a minimally invasive fashion during placement of pedicle screws, further gains in segmental lordosis can be achieved (**Fig. 5**).[12,13,20,21] A summary of

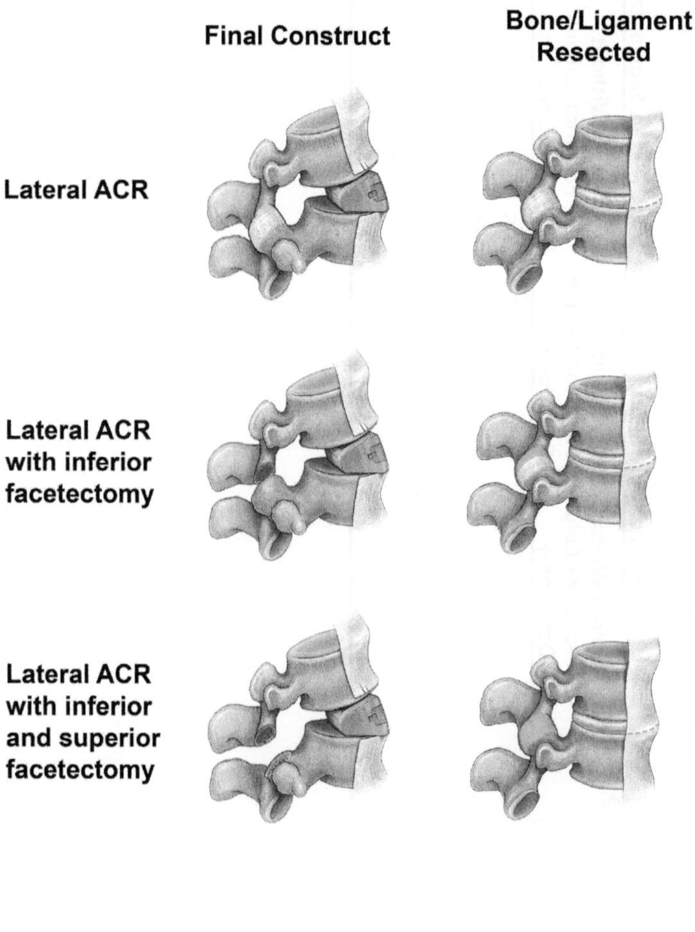

Final Construct   **Bone/Ligament Resected**

Lateral ACR

Lateral ACR with inferior facetectomy

Lateral ACR with inferior and superior facetectomy

Fig. 5. ACR with posterior osteotomies. Release of the ALL combined with varying posterior osteotomies can achieve greater segmental lordosis. The more destabilizing the posterior osteotomy, the greater the degree of segmental lordosis can be achieved at the index level of intervention. The left column of illustrations shows 3 ACR constructs with progressively greater segmental lordosis potential depending on the degree of posterior osteotomy. The right column illustrates the structures released and cut in green to achieve the desired ACR construct. (*Courtesy of* Barrow Neurological Institute, Phoenix, AZ.)

literature reported radiographic changes associated with ACR, with or without various osteotomies, is summarized in **Table 4**. Depending on the type of osteotomy performed as well as the implant used, the amount of lordosis restored by lateral ACR can match 3-column osteotomies at either a single treated level or through sequential adjacent treated levels with lower blood loss and incidence of major complications.[12,21,22]

Furthermore, the limited results reported to date from lateral ACR seem durable. The alignment achieved in the authors' patient cohort is maintained over 20-months of follow-up despite a 16.4% incidence of subsidence across all treated levels. All patients demonstrated a significant correction of their LL and reduction of their PI-LL mismatch, indicating sustainable spinopelvic harmony and improvement in sagittal balance. Thoracic hypokyphosis as a compensatory mechanism for positive sagittal balance also demonstrated a lasting improvement but did not reach statistical significance.

Morbidity

The MIS-LLIF approach for ACR remains novel, and the learning curve remains high. Devastating complications from injury to the great vessels, segmental vessels, and bowel have been described in the literature[23–25] but fortunately were not encountered in the authors' cohort. Because ACR builds on the same surgical workflow and initial approach as LLIF, there is a theoretic overlap of risks. Injury to the femoral nerve and lumbar plexus is one of the most serious neurologic risks associated with LLIF and may incur both sensory and motor deficits.

Unfortunately, wide inconsistencies exist within the literature with regard to reporting LLIF neurologic complications. Most studies provide inadequate details related to the anatomic source, severity of injury, and what type of LLIF technique was used or whether neuromonitoring, if any, was used. As a result, rates of sensory and motor deficits after LLIF have ranged wildly from 0.7% to 30% and from 3.4% to 23.7%, respectively.[26–29] Even when postoperative neurologic deficits do occur, more than 90% resolve spontaneously within a year.[27] Within the largest systematic case series examining the morbidity of LLIF, Rodgers and colleagues[26] treated 600 consecutive patients with the XLIF platform, including directional neuromonitoring, and reported a transient neurologic injury rate of only 0.7% with no incidence of any permanent neurologic deficits.

Lastly, placement of a large hyperlordotic cage may result in increased stress on the endplates, especially when combined with a posterior osteotomy, resulting in cage subsidence and loss of segmental correction. This process is likely responsible for the increased incidence of subsidence seen in the authors' treated disk space levels that underwent a posterior osteotomy but overall did not affect long-term radiographic outcomes.

Proximal Junctional Kyphosis

A recent meta-analysis reviewing 10 retrospective studies and 1230 patients undergoing open surgery for adult spinal deformity demonstrated a total radiographic PJK rate of 32.2%, with surgical rates of 6.7%.[17] This meta-analysis, however, incorporated multiple definitions of PJK, with criteria ranging from an absolute PJA of greater than 10° to as high as greater than 20° and a change in the PJA from greater than 5° to as high as greater than 20° as suggested in recent literature from the International Spine Study Group.[30,31] Consequently, the authors

Table 4
Overview of anterior column release segmental lordosis gains

Study	Type of Study	No. of Levels	Size of Interbody (°)	Segmental Lordosis Gained	Posterior Osteotomy
Present study	Clinical	26	30	11.7	None
Turner et al,[13] 2015	Clinical	24	20 and 30	9.9	None
Turner et al,[13] 2015	Clinical	7	30	15.4	Schwab 1
Present study	Clinical	29	30	17.3	Schwab 1
Melikian et al,[20] 2016	Cadveric biomechanical	13	30	10.5	Schwab 1
Melikian et al,[20] 2016	Cadveric biomechanical	13	30	26	Schwab 2
Turner et al,[13] 2015	Clinical	27	20 and 30	18.2	Schwab 2
Berjano et al,[12] 2015	Clinical	12	30	26	Schwab 2
Akbarnia et al,[21] 2014	Clinical	15	30	35	Schwab 2

chose to represent PJK rates by both the most stringent and most lenient definitions available for adequate integration into the spinal deformity literature.

The authors' overall PJK rates of 37% and 9.7%, by the most stringent and least stringent PJK definitions, respectively, are surprisingly in line with the incidence seen in open deformity correction surgeries. These findings suggest that the underlying pathophysiology driving PJK may be independent from local anatomic factors related to the surgical approach. Several biomechanical studies suggest that the most significant contributor to increased load and stress of spinal segments adjacent to an instrumented construct is the rigidity of the instrumentation.[32–34] Clearly, continued progress is needed to examine causes and preventative strategies for PJK, beginning with a unified radiographic definition.

Limitations

The retrospective nature of this study, low number of patients, and mean follow-up time are flaws with well-known associated weaknesses. Over time, progressive adoption of the ACR technique will increase the available sample size of patients with more substantial follow-up. Furthermore, to facilitate communication regarding ACR techniques, surgical planning, and patient outcomes, a unified classification system for ACR that considers the approach and supplementation with posterior osteotomies is warranted.

SUMMARY

Lateral ACR via an MIS-LLIF approach is a powerful surgical strategy for restoring LL in the treatment of adult spinal deformities. Coupled with different posterior osteotomies, lateral ACR allows manipulation of all 3 spinal columns and can achieve deformity correction metrics equivalent to traditional open 3-column osteotomies in a minimally invasive platform. These results expand the adult spinal deformity patient population that prior to the development of ACR was untreatable by MIS strategies.[35] Additional investigation is warranted regarding the incidence of PJK, interbody subsidence, and overall durability of radiographic outcomes.

REFERENCES

1. Ames CP, Smith JS, Scheer JK, et al. Impact of spinopelvic alignment on decision making in deformity surgery in adults: a review. J Neurosurg Spine 2012; 16(6):547–64.

2. Diebo BG, Oren JH, Challier V, et al. Global sagittal axis: a step toward full-body assessment of sagittal plane deformity in the human body. J Neurosurg Spine 2016;25(4):494–9.

3. Michael AL, Loughenbury PR, Rao AS, et al. A survey of current controversies in scoliosis surgery in the United Kingdom. Spine 2012;37(18):1573–8.

4. Than KD, Park P, Fu KM, et al. Clinical and radiographic parameters associated with best versus worst clinical outcomes in minimally invasive spinal deformity surgery. J Neurosurg Spine 2016;25(1):21–5.

5. Glassman SD, Bridwell K, Dimar JR, et al. The impact of positive sagittal balance in adult spinal deformity. Spine 2005;30(18):2024–9.

6. Schwab F, Lafage V, Patel A, et al. Sagittal plane considerations and the pelvis in the adult patient. Spine 2009;34(17):1828–33.

7. Schwab F, Blondel B, Chay E, et al. The comprehensive anatomical spinal osteotomy classification. Neurosurgery 2014;74(1):112–20 [discussion: 120].

8. Deukmedjian AR, Dakwar E, Ahmadian A, et al. Early outcomes of minimally invasive anterior longitudinal ligament release for correction of sagittal imbalance in patients with adult spinal deformity. ScientificWorldJournal 2012;2012:789698.

9. Uribe JS, Smith DA, Dakwar E, et al. Lordosis restoration after anterior longitudinal ligament release and placement of lateral hyperlordotic interbody cages during the minimally invasive lateral transpsoas approach: a radiographic study in cadavers. J Neurosurg Spine 2012;17(5):476–85.

10. Deukmedjian AR, Le TV, Baaj AA, et al. Anterior longitudinal ligament release using the minimally invasive lateral retroperitoneal transpsoas approach: a cadaveric feasibility study and report of 4 clinical cases. J Neurosurg Spine 2012;17(6):530–9.

11. Manwaring JC, Bach K, Ahmadian AA, et al. Management of sagittal balance in adult spinal deformity with minimally invasive anterolateral lumbar interbody fusion: a preliminary radiographic study. J Neurosurg Spine 2014;20(5):515–22.

12. Berjano P, Cecchinato R, Sinigaglia A, et al. Anterior column realignment from a lateral approach for the treatment of severe sagittal imbalance: a retrospective radiographic study. Eur Spine J 2015;24(Suppl 3):433–8.

13. Turner JD, Akbarnia BA, Eastlack RK, et al. Radiographic outcomes of anterior column realignment for adult sagittal plane deformity: a multicenter analysis. Eur Spine J 2015;24(Suppl 3):427–32.

14. Saigal R, Mundis GM Jr, Eastlack R, et al. Anterior column realignment (ACR) in adult sagittal deformity correction: technique and review of the literature. Spine 2016;41(Suppl 8):S66–73.

15. Mummaneni PV, Shaffrey CI, Lenke LG, et al. The minimally invasive spinal deformity surgery

algorithm: a reproducible rational framework for decision making in minimally invasive spinal deformity surgery. Neurosurg Focus 2014;36(5):E6.

16. Pimenta L. Lateral endoscopic transpsoas retroperitoneal approach for lumbar spine surgery. Paper presented at: VIII Brazilian Spine Society Meeting May 4, 2001, Belo Horizonte (Brazil).

17. Luo M, Wang P, Wang W, et al. Upper thoracic versus lower thoracic as site of upper-instrumented vertebrae for long fusion surgery in adult spinal deformity: a meta-analysis of proximal junctional kyphosis. World Neurosurg 2017;102:200–8.

18. Berjano P, Aebi M. Pedicle subtraction osteotomies (PSO) in the lumbar spine for sagittal deformities. Eur Spine J 2015;24(1):49–57.

19. Diebo BG, Lafage V, Varghese JJ, et al. After 9 years of 3-column osteotomies, are we doing better? Performance curve analysis of 573 surgeries with 2-year follow-up. Neurosurgery 2017. [Epub ahead of print].

20. Melikian R, Yoon ST, Kim JY, et al. Sagittal plane correction using the lateral transpsoas approach: a biomechanical study on the effect of cage angle and surgical technique on segmental lordosis. Spine 2016;41(17):E1016–21.

21. Akbarnia BA, Mundis GM Jr, Moazzaz P, et al. Anterior column realignment (ACR) for focal kyphotic spinal deformity using a lateral transpsoas approach and ALL release. J Spinal Disord Tech 2014;27(1):29–39.

22. Mundis GM Jr, Turner JD, Kabirian N, et al. Anterior column realignment has similar results to pedicle subtraction osteotomy in treating adults with sagittal plane deformity. World Neurosurg 2017;105:249–56.

23. Murray G, Beckman J, Bach K, et al. Complications and neurological deficits following minimally invasive anterior column release for adult spinal deformity: a retrospective study. Eur Spine J 2015;24(Suppl 3):397–404.

24. Uribe JS, Deukmedjian AR. Visceral, vascular, and wound complications following over 13,000 lateral interbody fusions: a survey study and literature review. Eur Spine J 2015;24(Suppl 3):386–96.

25. Mummaneni PV, Park P, Fu KM, et al. Does minimally invasive percutaneous posterior instrumentation reduce risk of proximal junctional kyphosis in adult spinal deformity surgery? A propensity-matched cohort analysis. Neurosurgery 2016;78(1):101–8.

26. Rodgers WB, Gerber EJ, Patterson J. Intraoperative and early postoperative complications in extreme lateral interbody fusion: an analysis of 600 cases. Spine (Phila Pa 1976) 2011;36(1):26–32.

27. Cummock MD, Vanni S, Levi AD, et al. An analysis of postoperative thigh symptoms after minimally invasive transpsoas lumbar interbody fusion. J Neurosurg Spine 2011;15(1):11–8.

28. Knight RQ, Schwaegler P, Hanscom D, et al. Direct lateral lumbar interbody fusion for degenerative conditions: early complication profile. J Spinal Disord Tech 2009;22(1):34–7.

29. Berjano P, Langella F, Damilano M, et al. Fusion rate following extreme lateral lumbar interbody fusion. Eur Spine J 2015;24(Suppl 3):369–71.

30. Scheer JK, Osorio JA, Smith JS, et al. Development of validated computer-based preoperative predictive model for proximal junction failure (PJF) or clinically significant PJK with 86% accuracy based on 510 ASD patients with 2-year follow-up. Spine 2016;41(22). E1328–e1335.

31. Smith JS, Shaffrey CI, Klineberg E, et al. Complication rates associated with 3-column osteotomy in 82 adult spinal deformity patients: retrospective review of a prospectively collected multicenter consecutive series with 2-year follow-up. J Neurosurg Spine 2017;27(4):444–57.

32. Bastian L, Lange U, Knop C, et al. Evaluation of the mobility of adjacent segments after posterior thoracolumbar fixation: a biomechanical study. Eur Spine J 2001;10(4):295–300.

33. Shono Y, Kaneda K, Abumi K, et al. Stability of posterior spinal instrumentation and its effects on adjacent motion segments in the lumbosacral spine. Spine 1998;23(14):1550–8.

34. Ha KY, Schendel MJ, Lewis JL, et al. Effect of immobilization and configuration on lumbar adjacent-segment biomechanics. J Spinal Disord 1993;6(2):99–105.

35. Haque RM, Mundis GM Jr, Ahmed Y, et al. Comparison of radiographic results after minimally invasive, hybrid, and open surgery for adult spinal deformity: a multicenter study of 184 patients. Neurosurg Focus 2014;36(5):E13.

Navigation-Assisted Minimally Invasive Surgery Deformity Correction

Taemin Oh, MD[a],*, Paul Park, MD[b],
Catherine A. Miller, MD[a], Andrew K. Chan, MD[a],
Praveen V. Mummaneni, MD[a]

KEYWORDS

- Deformity • Spine surgery • Navigation • Minimally invasive • Scoliosis

KEY POINTS

- Use of intraoperative navigation can be an important tool for minimally invasive surgery (MIS) deformity correction.
- In the circumferential MIS approach, deformity correction is typically broken down to 2 stages: stage 1 often involves a prepsoas or transpsoas lateral approach or anterior lumbar interbody fusion, whereas stage 2 involves MIS transforaminal lateral interbody fusion (if appropriate) with percutaneous screw instrumentation.
- Outcomes using navigation in MIS deformity correction have both shown to be successful when appropriate indications are followed.

INTRODUCTION

Minimally invasive approaches to spinal surgery (minimally invasive surgery [MIS]) offer a promising alternative to open approaches, with emphasis placed on minimizing exposure-related morbidity (eg, blood loss, postoperative pain). However, this same minimal exposure can also limit direct visualization of the spinal anatomy. Although use of fluoroscopy can partially offset this disadvantage, use of fluoroscopy can also increase ionizing radiation exposure to the surgeon, staff, and patients. Intraoperative navigation can, thus, perform a critical role during MIS surgery, as it can facilitate

both safety and accuracy during highly complex surgical procedures while decreasing intraoperative radiation exposure.[1–5]

One of the most common MIS methodologies for treating deformity involves a 2-stage approach: (1) stage 1 consists of a MIS transpsoas lateral extreme lateral interbody fusion [XLIF]/ direct lateral interbody fusion [DLIF] or oblique prepsoas approach for interbody fusion or an anterior lateral interbody fusion (ALIF); (2) stage 2 consists of a posterior approach, which can either incorporate open techniques (hybrid procedure) or exclusively use MIS techniques, such as the MIS transforaminal

Disclosure Statement: Drs T. Oh, C.A. Miller, and A.K. Chan have no interests to disclose. Dr C.A. Miller has an AOSpine fellow's grant. Dr P. Park is a consultant to Globus, Medtronic, NuVasive, and Zimmer-Biomet and receives royalties from Globus. Dr P.V. Mummaneni is a consultant to DePuy Spine, Globus, and Stryker, with financial support provided by DePuy Spine, Thieme Publishing, Quality Medical Publishers, and Taylor Francis Publishers. He has honoraria from AOSpine, own stock in Spinicity/ISD, and has received grants from the ISSG, AOSpine, and NREF.
^a Department of Neurological Surgery, University of California San Francisco, 505 Parnassus Avenue, Room M779, San Francisco, CA 94143-0112, USA; ^b Department of Neurological Surgery, University of Michigan, 1500 East Medical Center Drive SPC 5338, Ann Arbor, MI 48109-5338, USA
* Corresponding author.
E-mail address: taemin.oh@ucsf.edu

Neurosurg Clin N Am 29 (2018) 439–451
https://doi.org/10.1016/j.nec.2018.03.002
1042-3680/18/Published by Elsevier Inc.

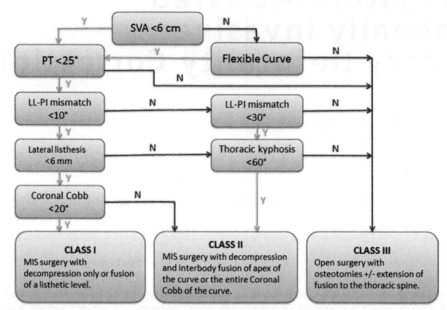

Fig. 1. Original MISDEF algorithm. LL-PI, lumbar lordosis-pelvic incidence; PT, pelvic tilt; SVA, sagittal vertical axis. (*From* Mummaneni PV, Shaffrey CI, Lenke LG, et al. The minimally invasive spinal deformity surgery algorithm: a reproducible rational framework for decision making in minimally invasive spinal deformity surgery. Neurosurg Focus 2014;36(5):E6; with permission.)

lateral interbody fusion (TLIF) with percutaneous instrumentation (circumferential MIS [cMIS]). The Minimally Invasive Spinal Deformity Surgery (MIS-DEF) algorithm can be used to assist in determining whether a cMIS approach is appropriate (**Fig. 1**).[6] In this article, the authors detail the use of navigation within the framework of a 2-stage approach (**Table 1**).

TYPICAL INDICATIONS/CONTRAINDICATIONS FOR LUMBAR FUSION USING NAVIGATION

See **Table 2**.

SURGICAL TECHNIQUE/PROCEDURE
Preoperative Planning

- Assessment of 36-in-long cassette radiographs is essential to characterize the degree of spinal curvature and deformity. Bending radiographs or supine computed tomography (CT) scouts with reformatted images are helpful to assess for flexibility and spinal instability.
- Fixed deformities are technically challenging to treat via cMIS, and the likelihood of suboptimal deformity correction is high. In such cases, a traditional open or hybrid approach should be considered unless advanced MIS techniques, such as the MIS pedicle subtraction osteotomy, is planned.

Intraoperative Computed Tomography–Guided Navigation

- Several intraoperative CT-guided navigation systems are available, including the O-arm/STEALTH (**Fig. 2**; Medtronic Inc, Minneapolis,

Table 1 Surgical Approaches	
Approach	**Basic Description**
cMIS	Combination of a 2-stage approach emphasizing MIS techniques: • Stage 1: MIS transpsoas lateral or oblique prepsoas approach or ALIF for interbody fusion • Stage 2: Percutaneous pedicle screw instrumentation, with or without MIS TLIF
Hybrid	Combination of a 2-stage approach with mix of MIS and open techniques: • Stage 1: MIS transpsoas lateral or oblique prepsoas approach or ALIF for interbody fusion • Stage 2: open pedicle screw instrumentation
Open	Combination of a 2-stage approach with emphasis primarily on open techniques

Table 2
Indications and contraindications

Typical Indications	Contraindications

• Failure of conservative therapy (eg, physical therapy, steroid injections) and symptoms attributable to spinal deformity, as defined by
  ○ Abnormal spinopelvic parameters (eg, PT, PI-LL mismatch, SVA)
  ○ Significant coronal curvature or imbalance
• Spondylolisthesis refractory to conservative therapy
	• Fixed deformity, as assessed by bending/supine films or CT scout, when considering cMIS
	  ○ Includes previous multilevel instrumented fusion
	• Severe deformity (ie, PI-LL mismatch >30°), when considering cMIS
	• Severe osteoporosis (relative contraindication)
	• Previous bowel surgery, when considering a lateral or oblique retroperitoneal MIS approach (relative contraindication)

Abbreviations: PI-LL, pelvic incidence-lumbar lordosis; PT, pelvic tilt; SVA, sagittal vertical axis.

Minnesota), Airo mobile CT-based spinal navigation system (**Fig. 3**; Brainlab, Feldkirchen, Germany), and the Stryker spinal navigation platform (Stryker, Kalamazoo, Michigan).[7]

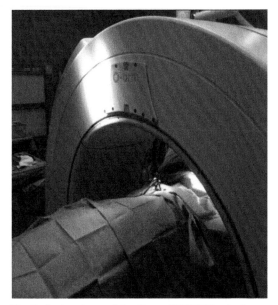

Fig. 2. Basic set-up of the O-arm/STEALTH spinal navigation system.

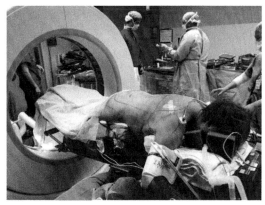

Fig. 3. Basic setup of the Airo Brainlab spinal navigation system.

- In principle, these systems use cone-beam CT technology to create a composite 360° 3-dimensional (3D) reconstruction of the patients' spine. Compared with non-navigated or fluoroscopy-based techniques, the benefits of CT-guided navigation include a high degree of fidelity for screw placement as well as reduced radiation exposure to the surgeon.[8–10]
- If applicable, the intraoperative CT scanner can be used to obtain an immediate postinstrumentation scan to verify accuracy if available.[11]

Technical notes

- In brief, patients are initially positioned on a Jackson table. A dynamic, percutaneous reference arc is secured in place; the location varies depending on the procedure (to be discussed in later sections).
- An intraoperative spin is performed on the relevant operative levels using a mobile, circular CT scanner. The composite 3D reconstruction data are exported to external software for navigation, and all the tools necessary for instrumentation can be calibrated and registered through an infrared reader.
- Anatomic landmarks can then be identified and verified to ensure registration accuracy. A dynamic monitor display provides real-time feedback to facilitate instrumentation and interbody fusion.[10–12]

Limitations

- Because registration is derived based on a fixed position of patients, any movement of patients or the reference frame can diminish accuracy. Care must especially be taken when applying any downward forces, such as when placing pedicle screws, as this can alter the spinal alignment.[11]

- Current navigation protocols do not allow for guidewire navigation. As a result, there is a risk of passing the guidewire too deep through the vertebral body and injuring intra-abdominal contents. To avoid this, the guidewire may be pulled back 1 to 2 cm once the proximal pedicle has been fully cannulated.[11] Alternatively, the Kirschner (K) wire can be bobbed up and down by 0.25 in during cannulation with the tap or screw placement in order to control its descent through the pedicle and avoid violating the ventral vertebral body (**Fig. 4**).

Stage 1: Lateral Transpsoas/Oblique Prepsoas Interbody Fusion

Anatomic planning considerations

- The iliac crest should be assessed via antero-posterior radiograph to determine if an orthogonal approach to the L4-5 disk space is feasible. A high-riding iliac crest would preclude the lateral transpsoas approach and necessitate use of the prepsoas approach.
- Assessment of the preoperative axial MRI is also critical, as anterior positioning of the psoas muscle at L4-5 is associated with more anterior positioning of the lumbar plexus (**Fig. 5**), which

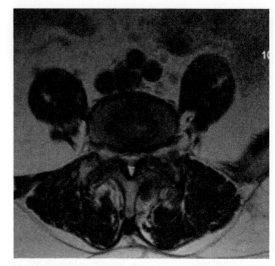

Fig. 5. Anterior position of the psoas muscle at L4-5.

translates to an increased theoretic risk of nerve plexus injury.
- Early aortic bifurcation can result in the iliac vessels crossing the anterolateral border of the L4-5 disk space, thereby increasing vascular injury risk with the prepsoas approach.
- Choosing between a concave versus convex approach is surgeon dependent, and at present there is no definitive evidence to support use of one over the other.

Prep and patient positioning

- Although not a universal practice, some surgeons advocate for bowel prep before surgery because of the rare risk of bowel injury.
- A radiolucent operating table is used, and the camera and navigation system are typically placed at the foot of the table. After attaching neuro-monitoring leads, patients are positioned in the lateral decubitus position. The authors prefer a left-sided approach, particularly for the prepsoas approach, because of the favorable iliac vein anatomy (**Fig. 6**).

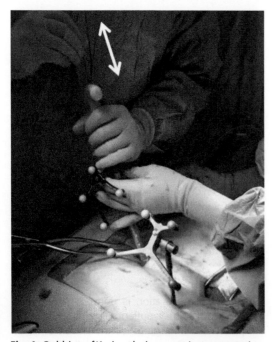

Fig. 4. Bobbing of K wires during screw instrumentation.

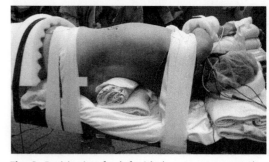

Fig. 6. Positioning for left-sided prepsoas approach.

- An axillary roll and flank roll are placed. The flank roll simulates breaking of the table and opens the space between the lower rib cage and iliac crest. The hip and knee are flexed to reduce tension on the psoas muscle. Patients are secured with tape at multiple points, and the skin is prepped and draped in standard fashion. Note: Fluoroscopy may not be used for preoperative localization if navigation is available.

Surgical approach

- A stab incision is made near the anterior superior iliac spine (ASIS) or alternatively near the posterior superior iliac spine (PSIS). Note that the sensory nerves (ilioinguinal, iliohypogastric nerves) run close to the ASIS; thus, care must be taken to avoid injury to these neural structures. An iliac pin is impacted into the bone. A navigation reference frame is attached (**Fig. 7**).
- Sterile drapes are applied. The intraoperative imaging unit is then used to obtain a 3D reconstructed image of the targeted spinal levels, which is then auto-registered to the navigation system. Typically, up to 4 spinal levels can be navigated after a single 3D image acquisition from the intraoperative imaging unit. The authors recommend starting with the disk level most distant from the frame.
- The incision site is determined using the navigation pointer with trajectory views to obtain an orthogonal or oblique approach to the targeted disk level. The incision is made followed

by dissection through the subcutaneous tissues until the abdominal wall musculature is identified. A muscle-splitting approach is used to enter the retroperitoneal space. For the prepsoas approach, the psoas muscle is swept posteriorly to the disk.
- A removable tracking frame is attached to the initial dilator. A clip electrode is also attached to this dilator for nerve stimulation (**Fig. 8**). Using navigation, the dilator is advanced through the psoas muscle into the midpoint of the targeted disk space for the transpsoas approach (**Fig. 9**). For the prepsoas approach, the dilator is advanced into the disk space in front of or through the anterior border of the psoas muscle (**Fig. 10**).
- Once the dilator is anchored onto the disk, sequential dilation is performed. A tubular retractor is placed. Positioning of the retractor and trajectory are assessed using the navigated dilator.

Surgical procedure

- A bayonetted knife is used to open the annulus. For collapsed disks, a navigated

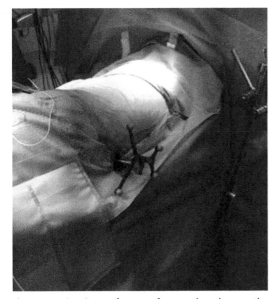

Fig. 7. Navigation reference frame placed near the PSIS.

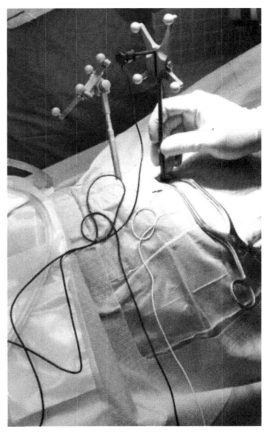

Fig. 8. Clip electrode attachment to navigated dilator.

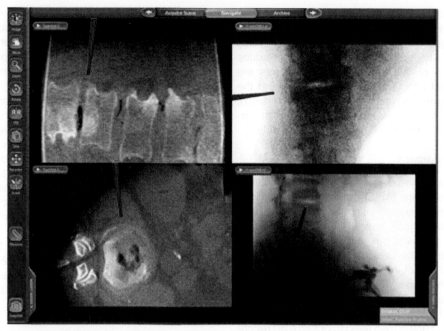

Fig. 9. Advancement of dilator through psoas muscle.

cobb is used instead to provide initial distraction. Discectomy is performed using various instruments, including rongeurs and navigated rotate shavers. Contralateral annular release is accomplished using the navigated cobb. Navigated cage trials are then used to determine the appropriate cage size (**Fig. 11**). The cage is filled with graft material and impacted into the disk space under navigation (**Fig. 12**).

- Many types of cages exist, including hyperlordotic and expandable options that may potentially improve segmental lordosis. As reported by Anand and colleagues,[1] hyperlordotic

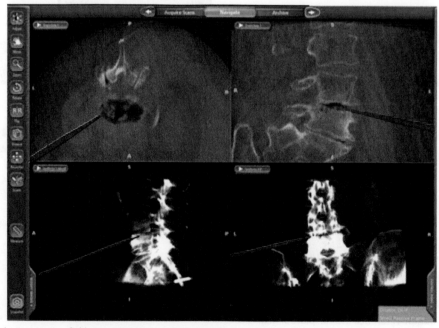

Fig. 10. Advancement of dilator anterior to psoas muscle.

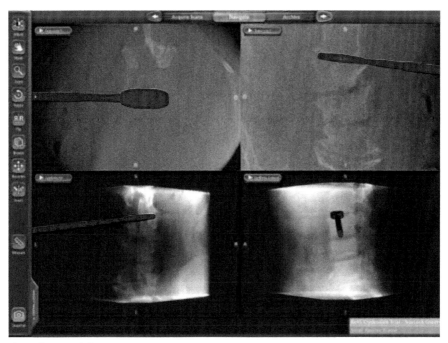

Fig. 11. Navigated cage trials.

cages (12°) are helpful in order to avoid having to release the anterior longitudinal ligament. However, one caveat to this would be that oversized cages may subside and result in loss of segmental lordosis.

- Use of fluoroscopy is minimized. With the authors' current experience, fluoroscopy is often used after navigated cage placement to confirm positioning. However, early in one's experience using navigation, fluoroscopy

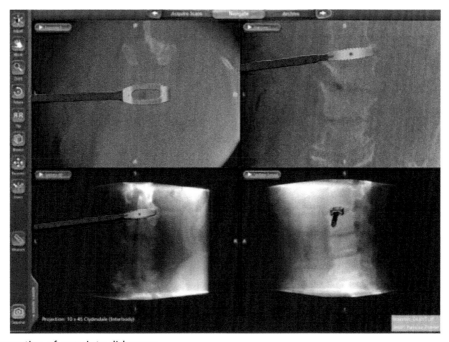

Fig. 12. Impaction of cage into disk space.

may be used more frequently for confirmation. In addition, for severely collapsed disk spaces where an osteotome is needed to enter the disk space, use of confirmatory fluoroscopy is recommended, as navigation does not provide enough accuracy to consistently preserve the end plate.

- If a fusion is required at the L5-S1 disk space, the prepsoas approach can be used with patients remaining in the same position.

Stage 2: Posterior Minimally Invasive Surgery Transforaminal Lateral Interbody Fusion and Percutaneous Pedicle Screws

Prep and patient positioning

- Similar to stage 1, a radiolucent flat Jackson table is used. A Wilson frame can be used to facilitate access to the disk space but should be lowered into lordosis before securing the rods. The navigation camera and monitor are typically placed at the foot of the table.
- Once neuro-monitoring leads are placed, patients are positioned prone with arms in super-man position. Patients are secured with tape at multiple points and padded accordingly. The skin is prepped and draped in standard fashion. Again, fluoroscopy is not needed for localization given the use of navigation.

Surgical approach

- A stab incision is made overlying the lower PSIS. The iliac pin is impacted into the bone with the tip angled laterally and superiorly so that the reference frame faces away from the operative field.[13] A layer of sterile draping is applied followed by 3D image acquisition by the intraoperative imaging unit.
- After auto-registration to the navigation system, the incision sites are determined by using the navigation pointer with trajectory views. Incision type, midline versus multiple paramedian, depends on surgeon preference. Midline incisions are sometimes needed if decompression is planned, and the reference arc can be placed on an exposed spinous process in such cases.[14]
- If a MIS-TLIF is planned, then it is performed first. Analogous to the lateral interbody fusion, the navigated initial dilator is advanced through the muscle orthogonal to the target disk space. Note: The reference arc is typically placed on the PSIS contralateral to the planned TLIF in order to avoid bumping the arc with the TLIF instruments.[15]

- Sequential dilation is performed with placement of the bladed retractor, which is then fixated into place with a table-mounted system. Positioning and trajectory of the retractor can be confirmed with the navigation pointer.

Surgical procedure

- Laminotomy, facetectomy, and discectomy are performed in the standard manner for TLIF.[16] After graft placement, the cage is impacted into the disk space under navigation guidance.
- Note: Intermittent fluoroscopy can be a helpful tool at this stage to visualize the degree of distraction and end plate preservation. The final position of the interbody device can also be confirmed with final fluoroscopy.[15]
- After cage placement, a second 3D image acquisition is often performed before screw placement to confirm cage placement and to reregister the spinal anatomy. As an alternative to obtaining multiple 3D image acquisitions, the MIS-TLIF can be performed under fluoroscopy only.
- For navigated screw placement, the number of instrumented levels will dictate the number of 3D image acquisitions needed. In general, 4 spinal segments can be imaged per acquisition.
- Attention is turned to the most proximal pedicle. The incision site is determined by the use of the navigation pointer. After incision, the underlying fascia is opened with a bovie cautery. A navigated awl-tap is advanced through the paraspinous muscles to dock on the bone in line with the pedicle (**Fig. 13**).
- The awl-tap is advanced through the pedicle into the vertebral body guided by navigation. The screw trajectory and positioning are saved in the navigation software so that the pedicle track can be located for final screw placement. Appropriate screw diameter and length can be determined by changing the size of the screw image on the navigation monitor.
- An appropriately sized minimally invasive pedicle screw with extended screw tabs is attached to a navigated screwdriver (**Fig. 14**). The screw is then inserted into the pedicle screw track previously created by the awl-tap guided by navigation (**Fig. 15**). This process is repeated on the contralateral side and appropriate spine levels.
- In cases of short-segment instrumentation (1–3 levels), the percutaneous incisions may be

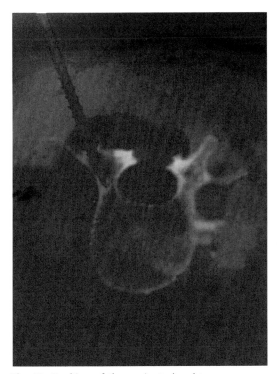

Fig. 13. Docking of the navigated awl-tap.

connected to facilitate rod insertion. In cases requiring 4 or more levels of fixation, MIS reduction towers can be docked and the rods placed under fluoroscopic guidance. Use of K wires is optional.[14]

- A rod is contoured and inserted through the extended screw tabs on the convex side of the curve (**Fig. 16**). The rod is rotated for lordosis. Set screws are placed sequentially. The rod holder is released. A second rod is contoured and inserted through the extended screw tabs on the contralateral side. Set screws are subsequently placed.

Complications and Management

- Complications associated with navigation are typically due to registration error or inadvertent movement of the reference frame. It is recommended that accuracy be verified periodically.
- Beyond those complications typically associated with spinal surgery (eg, infection), complications specifically associated with the MIS transpsoas interbody fusion include bowel injury, ureteral/renal injury, femoral nerve injury, vascular injury, pseudohernia (paresis of abdominal musculature), incisional hernias, and subsidence.

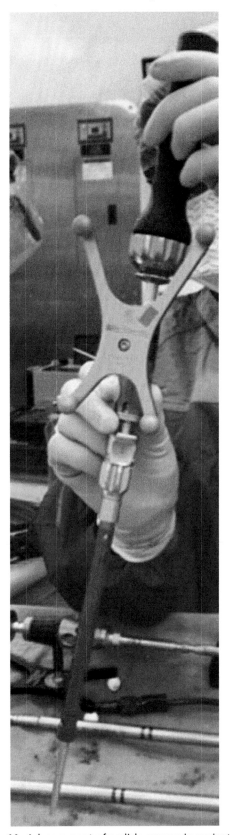

Fig. 14. Advancement of pedicle screws via navigated screwdriver.

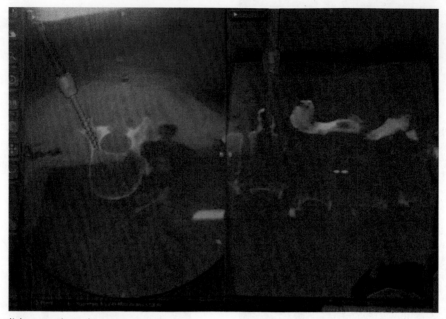

Fig. 15. Pedicle screw insertion.

Postoperative Care

- In general, principles of postoperative care for patients with deformity are similar regardless of whether MIS or open techniques are used.
- In the immediate postoperative period, serial blood count checks can be performed if there

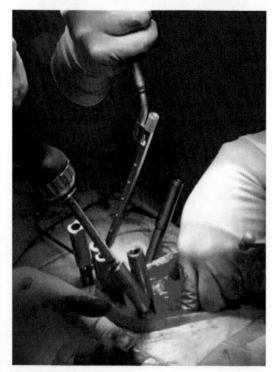

Fig. 16. Rod insertion.

is concern for unexpected intraoperative blood loss. Repletion is recommended, although the thresholds for doing so are surgeon dependent.

- Pain control is typically initiated using a patient-controlled analgesia pump for approximately 1 to 2 days and then tapered to intravenous pain medication and then oral medication. Nonsteroidal antiinflammatory drugs are avoided to minimize bleeding risks and to avoid pseudoarthrosis.
- Urinary catheters are usually removed on postoperative day 1.
- Aggressive bowel regimens should be implemented to facilitate bowel movement.
- Postoperative 3-ft-long cassette radiographs are obtained before discharge.

OUTCOMES

- Use of the minimally invasive transpsoas and prepsoas approaches in deformity surgery has been shown to be effective.[3,17,18] However, studies specifically focusing on these approaches with navigation guidance in deformity surgery are more limited.
- Initial investigations have shown that navigation-assisted transpsoas interbody fusion is feasible, accurate, and safe.[19–21] Zhang and colleagues[22] also showed significantly decreased radiation to the surgeon with the use of navigation for the prepsoas technique. Similarly, Liu and colleagues[23]

observed a decrease in radiation exposure to the surgeon and staff with use of navigation for the traditional transpsoas approach

- In most studies detailing the utility of navigation-guided deformity correction, the primary end point has been assessing the accuracy in placement of pedicle screws.[8,24–30] Within MIS deformity surgery, overall the results have indicated comparable efficacy with open, free-handed techniques.[7,12,14,31] In a series by Kim and colleagues,[14] the investigators placed 290 pedicle screws in a cohort of 48 adult patients and achieved a success rate of 96.6% without pedicle breach. Statistically significant improvements in clinical performance were noted, and no complications were observed or revision surgeries required. In a small study of 36 patients, of whom only 14 were treated for deformity, Smith and colleagues[32] reported no pedicle breaches based on radiography analysis and a 98.3% accuracy in patients with postoperative CT after MIS navigated pedicle screw placement. Zhu and colleagues[12] compared the efficacy of MIS with navigation with open approaches for correction of Lenke type 5C adolescent idiopathic scoliosis. Among 15 patients and 30 patients treated with MIS versus open approaches, respectively, their study revealed a similar degree of deformity correction and instrumentation accuracy. Morbidity (estimated blood loss, operative time, pain) was significantly less observed in the MIS cohort as well. Several large meta-analyses have corroborated these findings.[33–35]
- Hamilton and colleagues[36] published a series comparing MIS lateral interbody fusion with percutaneous pedicle instrumentation compared with hybrid versus open procedures and found that although the most common reason for reoperation in the MIS cohort was pseudoarthrosis, patients in this cohort were not at an increased risk for revision surgery compared with the others. Importantly, MIS techniques have also shown to result in similar clinical outcomes as the open and hybrid surgery groups.[37]

SUMMARY

Surgical correction of spinal deformity is a highly challenging endeavor associated with serious complications and the risk of negatively impacting patients' quality of life.[38–40] Recently, the adoption of minimally invasive techniques has been increasingly investigated as a means of reducing the likelihood of complications and morbidity while optimizing clinical and radiographic outcomes at the long-term follow-up.[1–5] Although use of intraoperative navigation is not a uniformly adopted protocol, with some investigators arguing against its routine use because of the increased radiation exposure,[4] navigation serves as an important adjunct that can be used based on the complexity of the surgery or patient anatomy.

REFERENCES

1. Anand N, Kong C, Fessler RG. A staged protocol for circumferential minimally invasive surgical correction of adult spinal deformity. Neurosurgery 2017; 81(5):733–9.
2. Eastlack RK, Mundis GM Jr, Wang M, et al. Is there a patient profile that characterizes a patient with adult spinal deformity as a candidate for minimally invasive surgery? Global Spine J 2017;7(7): 703–8.
3. Park HY, Ha KY, Kim YH, et al. Minimally invasive lateral lumbar interbody fusion for adult spinal deformity: clinical and radiological efficacy with minimum two years follow-up. Spine (Phila Pa 1976) 2017. [Epub ahead of print].
4. de Bodman C, Miyanji F, Borner B, et al. Minimally invasive surgery for adolescent idiopathic scoliosis: correction of deformity and peri-operative morbidity in 70 consecutive patients. Bone Joint J 2017;99-B(12):1651–7.
5. Than KD, Mummaneni PV, Bridges KJ, et al. Complication rates associated with open versus percutaneous pedicle screw instrumentation among patients undergoing minimally invasive interbody fusion for adult spinal deformity. Neurosurg Focus 2017;43(6):E7.
6. Mummaneni PV, Shaffrey CI, Lenke LG, et al. The minimally invasive spinal deformity surgery algorithm: a reproducible rational framework for decision making in minimally invasive spinal deformity surgery. Neurosurg Focus 2014;36(5):E6.
7. Overley SC, Cho SK, Mehta AI, et al. Navigation and robotics in spinal surgery: where are we now? Neurosurgery 2017;80(3S):S86–99.
8. Jin M, Liu Z, Liu X, et al. Does intraoperative navigation improve the accuracy of pedicle screw placement in the apical region of dystrophic scoliosis secondary to neurofibromatosis type I: comparison between O-arm navigation and free-hand technique. Eur Spine J 2016;25(6):1729–37.
9. Grelat M, Zairi F, Quidet M, et al. Assessment of the surgeon radiation exposure during a minimally invasive TLIF: comparison between fluoroscopy and O-arm system. Neurochirurgie 2015;61(4):255–9 [in French].
10. Oertel MF, Hobart J, Stein M, et al. Clinical and methodological precision of spinal navigation

assisted by 3D intraoperative O-arm radiographic imaging. J Neurosurg Spine 2011;14(4):532–6.

11. Kim TT, Johnson JP, Pashman R, et al. Minimally invasive spinal surgery with intraoperative image-guided navigation. Biomed Res Int 2016;2016: 5716235.

12. Zhu W, Sun W, Xu L, et al. Minimally invasive scoliosis surgery assisted by O-arm navigation for Lenke type 5C adolescent idiopathic scoliosis: a comparison with standard open approach spinal instrumentation. J Neurosurg Pediatr 2017;19(4): 472–8.

13. Baaj AA, Beckman J, Smith DA. O-Arm-based image guidance in minimally invasive spine surgery: technical note. Clin Neurol Neurosurg 2013;115(3): 342–5.

14. Kim TT, Drazin D, Shweikeh F, et al. Clinical and radiographic outcomes of minimally invasive percutaneous pedicle screw placement with intraoperative CT (O-arm) image guidance navigation. Neurosurg Focus 2014;36(3):E1.

15. Safaee MM, Oh T, Pekmezci M, et al. Radiation exposure with hybrid image-guidance-based minimally invasive transforaminal lumbar interbody fusion. J Clin Neurosci 2018;48:122–7.

16. Mummaneni PV, Rodts GE Jr. The mini-open transforaminal lumbar interbody fusion. Neurosurgery 2005;57(4 Suppl):256–61 [discussion: 256–61].

17. Ohtori S, Mannoji C, Orita S, et al. Mini-open anterior retroperitoneal lumbar interbody fusion: oblique lateral interbody fusion for degenerated lumbar spinal kyphoscoliosis. Asian Spine J 2015;9(4):565–72.

18. Bae J, Theologis AA, Strom R, et al. Comparative analysis of 3 surgical strategies for adult spinal deformity with mild to moderate sagittal imbalance. J Neurosurg Spine 2018;28(1):40–9.

19. Park P. Three-dimensional computed tomography-based spinal navigation in minimally invasive lateral lumbar interbody fusion: feasibility, technique, and initial results. Neurosurgery 2015;11(Suppl 2): 259–67.

20. Joseph JR, Smith BW, Patel RD, et al. Use of 3D CT-based navigation in minimally invasive lateral lumbar interbody fusion. J Neurosurg Spine 2016;25(3): 339–44.

21. DiGiorgio AM, Edwards CS, Virk MS, et al. Stereotactic navigation for the prepsoas oblique lateral lumbar interbody fusion: technical note and case series. Neurosurg Focus 2017;43(2):E14.

22. Zhang YH, White I, Potts E, et al. Comparison perioperative factors during minimally invasive prepsoas lateral interbody fusion of the lumbar spine using either navigation or conventional fluoroscopy. Global Spine J 2017;7(7):657–63.

23. Liu X, Joseph JR, Smith BW, et al. Analysis of intraoperative cone-beam computed tomography combined with image guidance for lateral lumbar interbody fusion. Oper Neurosurg (Hagerstown) 2017. [Epub ahead of print].

24. Liu YJ, Tian W, Liu B, et al. Comparison of the clinical accuracy of cervical (C2-C7) pedicle screw insertion assisted by fluoroscopy, computed tomography-based navigation, and intraoperative three-dimensional C-arm navigation. Chin Med J (Engl) 2010;123(21):2995–8.

25. Ishikawa Y, Kanemura T, Yoshida G, et al. Clinical accuracy of three-dimensional fluoroscopy-based computer-assisted cervical pedicle screw placement: a retrospective comparative study of conventional versus computer-assisted cervical pedicle screw placement. J Neurosurg Spine 2010;13(5): 606–11.

26. Sugimoto Y, Ito Y, Tomioka M, et al. Clinical accuracy of three-dimensional fluoroscopy (IsoC-3D)-assisted upper thoracic pedicle screw insertion. Acta Med Okayama 2010;64(3):209–12.

27. Vissarionov S, Schroeder JE, Novikov SN, et al. The utility of 3-dimensional-navigation in the surgical treatment of children with idiopathic scoliosis. Spine Deform 2014;2(4):270–5.

28. Kosterhon M, Gutenberg A, Kantelhardt SR, et al. Navigation and image injection for control of bone removal and osteotomy planes in spine surgery. Oper Neurosurg (Hagerstown) 2017;13(2): 297–304.

29. Tormenti MJ, Kostov DB, Gardner PA, et al. Intraoperative computed tomography image-guided navigation for posterior thoracolumbar spinal instrumentation in spinal deformity surgery. Neurosurg Focus 2010;28(3):E11.

30. Larson AN, Polly DW Jr, Guidera KJ, et al. The accuracy of navigation and 3D image-guided placement for the placement of pedicle screws in congenital spine deformity. J Pediatr Orthop 2012;32(6):e23-9.

31. Houten JK, Nasser R, Baxi N. Clinical assessment of percutaneous lumbar pedicle screw placement using the O-arm multidimensional surgical imaging system. Neurosurgery 2012;70(4):990–5.

32. Smith BW, Joseph JR, Kirsch M, et al. Minimally invasive guidewireless, navigated pedicle screw placement: a technical report and case series. Neurosurg Focus 2017;43(2):E9.

33. Verma R, Krishan S, Haendlmayer K, et al. Functional outcome of computer-assisted spinal pedicle screw placement: a systematic review and meta-analysis of 23 studies including 5,992 pedicle screws. Eur Spine J 2010;19(3): 370–5.

34. Du JP, Fan Y, Wu QN, et al. Accuracy of pedicle screw insertion among 3 image-guided navigation systems: systematic review and meta-analysis. World Neurosurg 2017;109:24–30.

35. Shin BJ, James AR, Njoku IU, et al. Pedicle screw navigation: a systematic review and meta-analysis of perforation risk for computer-navigated versus freehand insertion. J Neurosurg Spine 2012;17(2):113–22.

36. Hamilton DK, Kanter AS, Bolinger BD, et al. Reoperation rates in minimally invasive, hybrid and open surgical treatment for adult spinal deformity with minimum 2-year follow-up. Eur Spine J 2016;25(8):2605–11.

37. Haque RM, Mundis GM Jr, Ahmed Y, et al. Comparison of radiographic results after minimally invasive, hybrid, and open surgery for adult spinal deformity: a multicenter study of 184 patients. Neurosurg Focus 2014;36(5):E13.

38. Riley MS, Bridwell KH, Lenke LG, et al. Health-related quality of life outcomes in complex adult spinal deformity surgery. J Neurosurg Spine 2018;28(2):194–200.

39. Jain A, Hassanzadeh H, Puvanesarajah V, et al. Incidence of perioperative medical complications and mortality among elderly patients undergoing surgery for spinal deformity: analysis of 3519 patients. J Neurosurg Spine 2017;27(5):534–9.

40. Nunez-Pereira S, Vila-Casademunt A, Domingo-Sàbat M, et al. Impact of early unanticipated revision surgery on health-related quality of life after adult spinal deformity. Spine J 2017. [Epub ahead of print].

Can Minimally Invasive Transforaminal Lumbar Interbody Fusion Create Lordosis from a Posterior Approach?

Neel Anand, MD*, Christopher Kong, MD

KEYWORDS

- Minimally invasive surgery • Transforaminal lumbar interbody fusion • Lordosis • Spine surgery

KEY POINTS

- Lordosis obtained with a minimally invasive Transforaminal Lumbar Interbody Fusion (TLIF) is comparable to that achieved with an open TLIF.
- The multiple available protocols for MIS TLIF contribute to the range of reported outcomes and successes with deformity correction.
- Regardless of the protocol chosen, steps critical to lordosis correction include maintaining the patient in a lordotic position while prone, avoiding endplate violation when preparing the disk space, maximizing disk space height with an interbody device, and placing the graft under the apophyseal ring.
- If high-magnitude (eg, >10°) lordosis correction is required, alternative interbody fusion methods or surgical procedures should be considered.

INTRODUCTION: NATURE OF THE PROBLEM

The transforaminal lumbar interbody fusion (TLIF) was first introduced by Harms and Rollinger in 1998.[1] The procedure was novel in its ability to allow for a 3-column fusion to be obtained through a unilateral, transforaminal corridor via a single posterior approach. Compared with its predecessor, the posterior lumbar interbody fusion, the TLIF required less retraction of the neural elements. This in turn resulted in a decreased rate of postoperative radiculitis.[2]

The TLIF has gained tremendous popularity among spine surgeons over the past 2 decades. This has exposed it to significant study, reworking, and evolution. Among the most significant enhancements of the procedure is its ability to be performed in a minimally invasive fashion. The term, *minimally invasive*, however, is nonspecific and has been applied equally to a variety of different protocols. As a result, reported outcomes for the MIS TLIF have been varied as well.[3–5]

One of the most highly scrutinized determinants of postoperative success after a TLIF is the restoration or improvement of lordosis. Failure to adequately address this goal can either perpetuate or lead to the development of flat back syndrome, where lumbar hypolordosis causes painful sagittal imbalance and increases the rate of adjacent segment degeneration.[6–11]

Disclosure Statement: Neel Anand, MD Royalties: Medtronics, Globus Medical, Elsevier Consultant: Medtronics Stocks: Globus Medical, Medtronics Stock Options: Paradigm Spine, Atlas Spine, Theracell, Bonovo Surgical.
Department of Orthopaedic Surgery, Cedars-Sinai Medical Center, 444 South San Vicente Boulevard, Suite 800, Los Angeles, CA 90048, USA
* Corresponding author.
E-mail address: neel.anand@cshs.org

Neurosurg Clin N Am 29 (2018) 453–459
https://doi.org/10.1016/j.nec.2018.03.010
1042-3680/18/© 2018 Elsevier Inc. All rights reserved.

Some MIS TLIF techniques have been shown capable of reproducibly inducing good lordosis correction.[4,12] One of those techniques is discussed in this article. Recent literature on other techniques that optimize lordosis when performing a TLIF is also reviewed. Variations in protocol or equipment that are not aimed at affecting lordosis, such as spacer material selection, are not discussed.

INDICATIONS/CONTRAINDICATIONS

Indications for the MIS TLIF are identical to those for open TLIF. These currently include symptomatic lumbar spondylolisthesis with or without neurologic symptoms, intractable pain from degenerative disease, and scoliosis.[13] An intervertebral disk space that is unable to accommodate distraction is considered a contraindication.[14]

Despite the deformity-correcting abilities of the TLIF, it has been described by many investigators that alternative interbody fusion methods can offer superior sagittal alignment correction. This includes anterior lumbar interbody fusion (ALIF) and lateral lumbar interbody fusion (LLIF). Both have been compared with the TLIF in multiple studies and found superior at inducing lordosis.[3,15,16]

Lumbar lordosis is seldom the only goal of surgery, however. There are, therefore, many circumstances under which a TLIF still presents itself as the best surgical option. Some of its advantages over other interbody fusion methods include decreased blood loss, cost, operative time, and complication rates.[17-19] The posterior approach allows for direct visualization and confirmation of neural decompression, while avoiding the abdominal organs and great vessels. Additionally, the unilateral placement of the cage combined with ipsilateral facetectomy is capable of imposing a coronal deformity correction superior to ALIF cages.[16]

One of the reasons that the TLIF remains so widely used today is that it is a versatile procedure. It can be performed with varying levels of resources, using open or minimally invasive techniques, and be easily incorporated into longer fusion constructs. This flexibility in technique has unfortunately led to significant inconsistencies in outcomes when reporting on postoperative lumbar lordosis.[4,12,20-22]

Some of the described advantages of MIS TLIF have been decreased postoperative radiculitis, hematoma formation, wound infection, and requirement for revision surgery.[12] Disadvantages have included increased radiation exposure to both patient and surgeon, learning curve, and requirement for special (bayonetted) instruments. Although not necessarily more common, cerebrospinal fluid leaks can also be more difficult to manage when performing an MIS TLIF.

SURGICAL TECHNIQUE/PROCEDURE
Preoperative Planning

The facetectomy is planned on the side with the more severe radiculopathy. Central and contralateral decompression can still be performed an MIS approach; thus, their necessity does not preclude the use of this technique. The MRI and CT are examined closely to identify anatomic variances, such as facet cysts, disk herniations, and pars fractures. Pedicle sizes are measured on cross-sectional imaging as well. If coronal deformity is identified on upright plain films, this can be used to dictate final placement of the interbody cage in the coronal plane. Severe osteoporosis identified on preoperative dual-energy x-ray absorptiometry scan should be corrected prior to surgery and managed postoperatively as well. In the setting of multilevel surgery or deformity correction involving long construct fusion, full-length upright scoliosis films are obtained. The spinopelvic and sagittal alignment parameters are calculated, and the accompanying corrective surgery/construct is planned.

Preparation, Positioning, and Equipment

The patient is positioned prone on a Jackson table. This table is preferred by the authors over a Wilson frame. Hips are maintained in extension. When positioned appropriately, the anterior superior iliac spine is freely palpable, proximal to the bolsters supporting the hips and thighs. Altogether, this helps to maximize a patient's lordosis on the operating table. Bony prominences are padded. Care is taken to avoid over-padding patients to the point where they are able to slip or lose position when the table is tilted intraoperatively. Other investigators have described using breaking Jackson tables to induce additional lordosis before final tightening of the posterior construct.[5,23] The authors have not found this necessary. Cases of fracture associated with table extension greater than 10° have been documented.[23]

The patient's operative site is draped wide to avoid introducing any draping material into the wound with percutaneous instruments.

A tubular retractor and microscope is used for the approach and exposure. Fluoroscopy is used for localization. Bayonetted, long instruments are required. For a single-level fusion, the authors typically use 5 mL of allograft demineralized bone matrix (DBM) putty and 4 mg of recombinant human bone morphogenetic protein-2 (rhBMP-2) (Infuse, Medtronics, Memphis, Tennessee).

Surgical Procedure

Step 1: localization and incisions
Fluoroscopy is used to confirm the levels of interest. Anterior-posterior (AP) shots orthogonal to the vertebral body are used to trace the lateral borders of the pedicles on the skin. The incision lines are drawn by connecting these traced lateral borders. For a single-level MIS TLIF, the incisions are typically 1-in long. Cautery is used to carry the exposures down to fascia and maintain hemostasis.

Step 2: pedicle canalization and wire placement
Jamshidi needles are introduced under fluoroscopic guidance into the pedicles. At L3, the starting point is at approximately the 3-o'clock position on the left side and the 9-o'clock position on the right side. More distally, the starting point is slightly more cephalad, and more proximal, the starting point is slightly more caudal. The Jamshidi needles are advanced until they are approximately 2 cm to 3 cm deep. In avoidance of medial breach, the tip of the needle should remain lateral to the medial pedicle border on the AP view. On lateral fluoroscopic views, once it is confirmed that the Jamshidi needles have traversed the full length of the pedicles, wires are placed through their cannulas. The free ends of the wires are then gently retracted away from the surgical field and secured to the drapes with forceps. An example of this is shown in **Fig. 1**. The fascia bridging the 2 wires on each side is released with cautery.

Step 3: exposure of the pars and facet
Under fluoroscopic guidance, sequential dilators are introduced onto the pars of the vertebra of interest. The first dilator is introduced in the muscular interval defined by the 2 previously placed guide wires. Sequential dilators are then placed over the first dilator until a retractable tubular dilator can be assembled. An example of a fully assembled tubular retractor is shown in **Fig. 2**. This is then secured to the operative table. Cautery is used to remove the remaining muscle fibers off of the lamina contained within the field of view. The pars and facet are visualized under microscopy.

Step 4: facetectomy and decompression
With the pars well defined, the inferior facet of the rostral vertebra is removed using a 0.25-in osteotome. The first cut is made transversely and the second cut is made more medially, parallel to the joint line. Prior to performing the first cut,

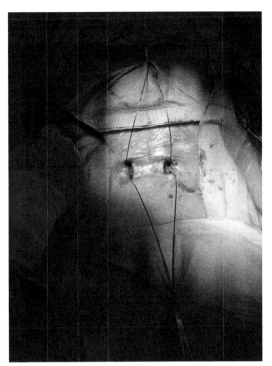

Fig. 1. The pedicles of the vertebrae above and below the level of interest are cannulated using Jamshidi needles. The needle stylettes are replaced with flexible guide wires that are retracted out of the field and held in place with forceps. The fascia bridging the 2 wires on either side is released with cautery.

the location of the osteotome is confirmed with lateral fluoroscopy. There should be adequate superior articular facet deep to the planned osteotomy before proceeding. If not, such as in the setting of a higher-grade spondylolisthesis, the inferior facetectomy can be performed with a high-speed bur. Once the inferior facet is removed, the decompression can be widened with the bur to better visualize the canal contents and lateral recess. The flavum is gradually excised. A medial portion of the superior facet is excised only insofar as it allows visibility of the lateral thecal sac, traversing nerve root shoulder and medial pedicle border. The exiting nerve root is not exposed. Excessive superior articular facet resection is avoided because this can weaken the superior cortex of its subadjacent pedicle, leading to fracture during interpedicular compression. After ipsilateral decompression to the lateral recess, the table, microscope, and tubular retractor can be tilted to access and decompress the central canal contralateral lateral recess and foramen if deemed necessary. Bone dust is collected as autograft whenever the high-speed bur is used.

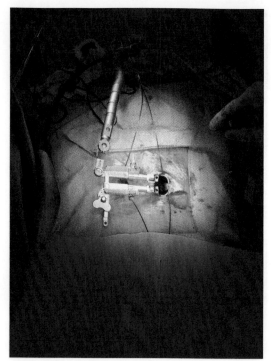

Fig. 2. After the fluoroscopically guided placement of sequential tubular dilators, an adjustable tubular retractor is placed into wound. This is introduced through the muscular interval defined by the guide wire above and below. The tubular retractor allows for visualization of the pars and facet. The lateral gap between its blades allows for intervertebral instruments to be directed more medially when levering handles laterally.

Step 5: diskectomy, endplate preparation, and interbody spacer placement

A box-cut annulotomy is performed using a 15 blade scalpel. A crude initial diskectomy is performed, using pituitary rongeurs and down-pushing curettes. This may require some gentle medial retraction of the thecal sac. The authors recommend avoiding constant retraction with a nerve root retractor. Instead, it is their preference to intermittently retract with a Frazier sucker tip when introducing an instrument into the disk space.

Once the lateral recess is free of compression from any disk bulging or herniation, an osteotome is placed over the superior lip of the caudal vertebral body. This bony lip is removed with the osteotome. Endplate preparation proceeds with continued use of the down-pushing curette, pituitaries, paddle shavers, rasps, and bayonetted curettes. Care is taken to avoid violating the endplates with the reaming instruments. Once the diskectomy is complete, residual loose disk material is evacuated by irrigating the disk space.

Trial spacers are then malleted into the disk space. A spacer with tight interference fit is selected as the final size.

A bullet-nosed, curved, steerable, polyetheretherketone static cage is assembled on the back table. The authors prefer to pack rhBMP-2 into the cage, surrounded by DBM putty. Placing rhBMP-2 posterior to the cage should be avoided, placing the rhBMP-2 anterior to the cage is acceptable. Under fluoroscopic guidance, the cage is malleted anteriorly until it reaches the anterior apophyseal ring. There, it is rotated until the entire cage is contained within the anterior third of the disk space. Autograft and additional DBM putty are then tightly packed behind the cage.

Step 6: posterior instrumentation and cantilever reduction

The pedicle wires are released from the drapes. Soft tissue dilators are placed over each wire. The pedicles are tapped over the wires. Cannulated screws with attached rod-reduction towers are then placed over each wire. Placement is confirmed with fluoroscopy. Wires are removed and precontoured rods are guided down the rod-reduction towers to the pedicle screw tulips. The caudal screw is reduced first, followed by the rostral screw. This reduction along the contoured rod helps to reduce the listhetic slip while also increasing lordosis. The maneuver is known as cantilever reduction. No additional interpedicular compression is applied.

As an added option for fusion, the contralateral facet can be exposed through the intermuscular interval established by the percutaneously placed screws. The facet interface can be decorticated with a high-speed bur and packed with rhBMP-2, autograft, and allograft. It has been the authors' experience over the past 5 years that this postero-lateral fusion using bone morphogenetic protein has not been necessary to reliably achieve fusion.

Step 7: final assessment and closure

Final AP and lateral fluoroscopic shots are taken. Images are closely scrutinized for aberrant screw placement or cage subsidence. The canal and bilateral foramina are palpated with a Woodson tool to rule out residual stenosis and remove any graft material that could have migrated. Meticulous hemostasis is obtained and the wound is closed in layers. Marcaine is injected into the muscle and subcutaneous tissues during closure. No drain is placed.

COMPLICATIONS AND MANAGEMENT

- Durotomy: direct repair, supplemented with fibrin glue

- Cage subsidence: prevent with meticulous preservation of the endplates
- Pedicle screw loss of purchase: upsize screw or convert to cortical screw
- Recurrent stenosis secondary to herniation of residual disk material or migration of bone graft material or rhBMP-2: prevent with thorough inspection and palpation of canal and foramina prior to closure
- Postoperative recurrent stenosis secondary to heterotopic ossification: prevent with maintaining rhBMP-2 in the anterior column of the disk space. If bony overgrowth is present, CT-navigated decompression can be performed.
- Anterior passage of instruments through the anterior longitudinal ligament when performing diskectomy: prevent with regular fluoroscopic images to verify location of instrument tips

POSTOPERATIVE CARE

- Patient is mobilized as soon as possible, often on the day of surgery.
- Depending on patients' health, they may be appropriate for discharge home on the day of surgery.
- No brace is required.
- Bone-strengthening medications, such as teriparatide, should be continued for patients with osteoporosis.
- Anti-inflammatory medications are avoided.

OUTCOMES

The results of this protocol have been previously published by the senior author of this article.[4] From 2002 through 2003, 100 patients were collected and subsequently followed for a minimum of 2 years. Average blood loss was

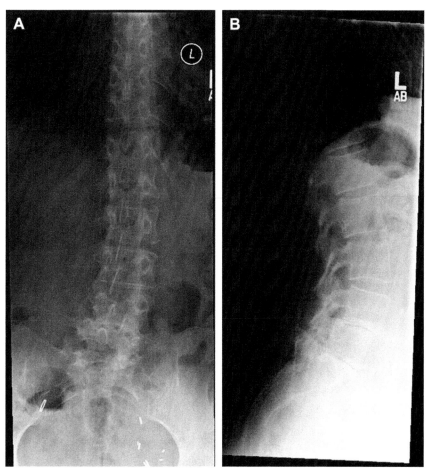

Fig. 3. Preoperative (A) AP and (B) lateral standing lumbar radiographs. Preoperative, standing lumbar radiographs of a 64-year-old woman with claudication and low back pain. Severe spondylosis with disk height loss is present at L4/L5 and L5/S1. There is anterolisthesis present at L4/L5. Segmental lumbar lordosis from L4 to S1 is 15°.

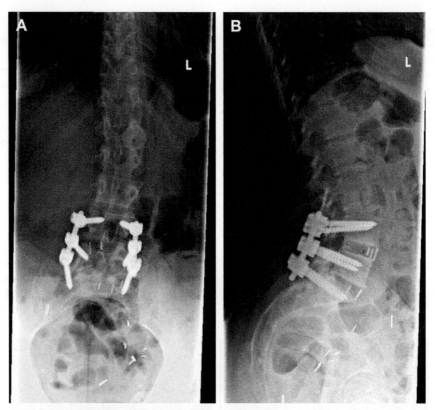

Fig. 4. Postoperative (*A*) AP and (*B*) lateral standing lumbar radiographs. A right-sided L4/L5 and a left-sided L5/S1 MIS TLIF have been performed. Segmental lordosis from L4 to S1 has increased to 41°.

300 mL. Average length of stay was 2.2 days. Pain scores reduced from an average of 9 (of 10) preoperative to an average of 3 at final follow-up. The average lordosis correction was 7°. The average anterior disk height increase was 8 mm. There were no cases of subsidence or screw malposition. Solid fusion was obtained in 99 of 100 patients.

The lordosis achieved with this method is comparable to what has been published for open TLIF techniques that also used bilateral facetectomies.[24,25]

CASE EXAMPLE

A 64-year-old woman presented with several years of worsening low back pain and neurogenic claudication affecting the bilateral lower extremities. She had failed nonoperative management. She was neurologically intact. Upright lumbar radiographs (shown in **Fig. 3**) revealed lumbar spondylosis with disk height loss at L4/L5 and L5/S1. A low-grade spondylolisthesis was present at L4/L5. Segmental lumbar lordosis in the region was 15°. An MRI (not shown) demonstrated severe central stenosis with left-sided foraminal stenosis at L5/S1 and right-sided foraminal

stenosis at L4/5L. The patient underwent a right-sided MIS TLIF at L4/L5 and a left-sided MIS TLIF at L5/S1. The cantilever reduction maneuver was used to increase local lordosis. Postoperative radiographs (**Fig. 4**) show a segmental lumbar lordosis of 41°.

SUMMARY

This article presents an MIS TLIF protocol that is capable of restoring lordosis as effectively as other available open TLIF techniques. If correction greater than 10° is indicated, an osteotomy, such as a Ponte, or pedicle subtraction should be considered in addition to or instead of the TLIF. As in open surgery, the crucial steps for successful lordosis correction when performing an MIS TLIF are maintaining the patient in a lordotic position while prone, avoiding endplate violation when preparing the disk space, maximizing disk space height with an interbody device, and placing the graft under the apophyseal ring.

REFERENCES

1. Harms J, Rolinger H. A one-stage procedure in operative treatment of spondylolistheses: dorsal

traction-reposition and anterior fusion. Z Orthop Ihre Grenzgeb 1982;120:343–7 (Ger).

2. Humphreys SC, Hodges SD, Patwardhan AG, et al. Comparison of posterior and transforaminal approaches to lumbar interbody fusion. Spine 2001; 26(5):567–71.

3. Lee N, Kim KN, Yi S, et al. Comparison of outcomes of anterior, posterior, and transforaminal lumbar interbody fusion surgery at a single lumbar level with degenerative spinal disease. World Neurosurg 2017;101:216–26.

4. Anand N, Hamilton JF, Perri B, et al. Cantilever TLIF with structural allograft and RhBMP2 for correction and maintenance of segmental sagittal lordosis: long-term clinical, radiographic, and functional outcome. Spine 2006;31(20):E748–53.

5. Hawasli AH, Khalifeh JM, Chatrath A, et al. Minimally invasive transforaminal lumbar interbody fusion with expandable versus static interbody devices: radiographic assessment of sagittal segmental and pelvic parameters. Neurosurg Focus 2017;43(2):E10–9.

6. Glassman SD, Bridwell K, Dimar JR, et al. The impact of positive sagittal balance in adult spinal deformity. Spine 2005;30(18):2024–9.

7. Lazennec JY, Ramaré S, Arafati N, et al. Sagittal alignment in lumbosacral fusion: relations between radiological parameters and pain. Eur Spine J 2000;9(1):47–55.

8. Recnik G, Košak R, Vengust R. Influencing segmental balance in isthmic spondylolisthesis using transforaminal lumbar interbody fusion. J Spinal Disord Tech 2013;26(5):246–51.

9. Kim S-B, Jeon T-S, Heo Y-M, et al. Radiographic results of single level transforaminal lumbar interbody fusion in degenerative lumbar spine disease: focusing on changes of segmental lordosis in fusion segment. Clin Orthop Surg 2009;1(4):207–13.

10. Moreau PE, Ferrero E, Riouallon G, et al. Radiologic adjacent segment degeneration 2 years after lumbar fusion for degenerative spondylolisthesis. Orthop Traumatol Surg Res 2016;102(6):759–63.

11. Yamasaki K, Hoshino M, Omori K, et al. Risk factors of adjacent segment disease after transforaminal inter-body fusion for degenerative lumbar disease. Spine 2017;42(2):E86–92.

12. Wong AP, Smith ZA, Stadler JA, et al. Minimally invasive transforaminal lumbar interbody fusion (MI-TLIF): surgical technique, long-term 4-year prospective outcomes, and complications compared with an open TLIF cohort. Neurosurg Clin N Am 2014;25(2): 279–304.

13. Jagannathan J, Sansur CA, Oskouian RJ Jr, et al. Radiographic restoration of lumbar alignment after transforaminal lumbar interbody fusion. Neurosurgery 2009;64(5):955–64.

14. Moskowitz A. Transforaminal lumbar interbody fusion. Orthop Clin North Am 2002;33(2):359–66.

15. Ajiboye RM, Alas H, Mosich GM, et al. Radiographic and clinical outcomes of anterior and transforaminal lumbar interbody fusions: a systematic review and meta analysis of comparative studies. Clin Spine Surg 2017. https://doi.org/10. 1097/BSD.0000000000000549.

16. Dorward IG, Lenke LG, Bridwell KH, et al. Transforaminal versus anterior lumbar interbody fusion in long deformity constructs. Spine 2013;38(12):E755–62.

17. Yang E-Z, Xu J-G, Liu X-K, et al. An RCT study comparing the clinical and radiological outcomes with the use of PLIF or TLIF after instrumented reduction in adult isthmic spondylolisthesis. Eur Spine J 2015;25(5):1587–94.

18. Jiang S-D, Chen J-W, Jiang L-S. Which procedure is better for lumbar interbody fusion: anterior lumbar interbody fusion or transforaminal lumbar interbody fusion? Arch Orthop Trauma Surg 2012;132(9): 1259–66.

19. Mobbs RJ, Phan K, Malham G, et al. Lumbar interbody fusion: techniques, indications and comparison of interbody fusion options including PLIF, TLIF, MI-TLIF, OLIF/ATP, LLIF and ALIF. J Spine Surg 2015;1(1):2–18.

20. Shen X, Wang L, Zhang H, et al. Radiographic analysis of one-level minimally invasive transforaminal lumbar interbody fusion (MI-TLIF) with unilateral pedicle screw fixation for lumbar degenerative diseases. Clin Spine Surg 2016;29(1):E1–8.

21. Lee W-C, Park J-Y, Kim KH, et al. Minimally invasive transforaminal lumbar interbody fusion in multilevel: comparison with conventional transforaminal interbody fusion. World Neurosurg 2016;85(C):236–43.

22. Hara M, Nishimura Y, Nakajima Y, et al. Transforaminal lumbar interbody fusion for lumbar degenerative disorders: mini-open TLIF and corrective TLIF. Neurol Med Chir (Tokyo) 2015;55(7):547–56.

23. Saville PA, Anari JB, Smith HE, et al. Vertebral body fracture after TLIF: a new complication. Eur Spine J 2016;25(Suppl 1):230–8.

24. Yson SC, Santos ERG, Sembrano JN, et al. Segmental lumbar sagittal correction after bilateral transforaminal lumbar interbody fusion. J Neurosurg Spine 2012;17(1):37–42.

25. Lindley TE, Viljoen SV, Dahdaleh NS. Effect of steerable cage placement during minimally invasive transforaminal lumbar interbody fusion on lumbar lordosis. J Clin Neurosci 2014;21(3):441–4.

Minimally Invasive Pedicle Subtraction Osteotomy

Andrew A. Fanous, MD, Jason I. Liounakos, MD, Michael Y. Wang, MD*

KEYWORDS

- Pedicle subtraction osteotomy • PSO • Minimally invasive surgery • MIS • Spinal deformity
- Scoliosis

KEY POINTS

- The prevalence of symptomatic adult spinal deformity is expected to continue to increase along with our ever-aging population. Although traditional open surgical techniques are effective at correcting spinal deformity, they are associated with high morbidity.
- Advantages of pedicle subtraction osteotomy (PSO) include the ability to treat a rigid spine, little restriction on the level of surgery, and lack of need to reposition the patient during surgery.
- The minimally invasive surgery (MIS) PSO strives to fulfill the objectives of MIS spine surgery, which include reduced intraoperative blood loss, soft tissue destruction, postoperative pain, and narcotic use while facilitating early mobilization.
- MIS PSO involves an exposure just wide enough to directly decompress and protect vital neural structures, while using a rod-cantilever technique to maximize lordosis.
- Preliminary evidence suggests MIS PSO results in good clinical outcomes with significant improvements in patient-reported outcomes as well as deformity correction.

INTRODUCTION

Adult spinal deformity (ASD) is a significant condition that affects the quality of life of thousands of people every year. With the substantially lengthened life span in the developed world, the prevalence of this condition is expected to increase markedly during the next few decades.[1] Many advances have been made and many new surgical techniques have been developed for the treatment of spinal deformity in both the sagittal and coronal planes. Open surgical techniques for the correction of kyphosis and/or scoliosis rely on osteotomies and/or restoration of anterior column height.[2–5] These open techniques, however, result in significant blood loss and a high rate of perioperative morbidity. The complication rate for such surgeries is at least 50% and can be as high as 90%, as shown in some large series.[6–8] The rate of major complications is significantly higher compared with that associated with their minimally invasive counterparts.[9] As such, there has been tremendous interest in the development, refinement, and study of less invasive techniques to achieve the same goals.

MINIMALLY INVASIVE SPINE SURGERY

To improve outcomes and minimize complications in ASD patients undergoing surgical correction, various minimally invasive surgical techniques have been developed over the past decade.[10] Studies have demonstrated, however, that there are limitations to using such techniques compared with open surgery. For instance, various reports describe an upper limit in the degree of coronal

Disclosure Statement: Dr M.Y. Wang serves as a consultant for and receives royalty payments from DePuy-Synthes Spine, Inc; is a consultant for Aesculap Spine; owns stock in Spinicity; and has received grants from the Department of Defense.
Department of Neurological Surgery, University of Miami, 1095 Northwest 14th Terrace, Miami, FL 33136, USA
* Corresponding author.
E-mail address: Mwang2@med.miami.edu

Neurosurg Clin N Am 29 (2018) 461–466
https://doi.org/10.1016/j.nec.2018.03.011

curvature correction possible using MIS techniques without exposure of the dorsal spine that would allow for multilevel open osteotomies.[9] In addition, MIS faces certain limitations with regard to improvement of lumbar lordosis and sagittal balance.[2,11] Today, the most common spine MIS procedure for ASD correction is lateral lumbar interbody fusion.[1] This technique results in minimal improvement in overall lumbar lordosis; however, that amounts to only 5° to 10° of correction.[11–13]

The development of anterior longitudinal ligament release to add lumbar lordosis represents a significant advancement in lateral MIS surgery and is covered in detail in other sections of this publication.[14] Although a powerful alternative to open surgery, there are limits to anterior column reconstruction MIS surgery. These include (1) the inability to treat already fused levels of the spine (requires a flexible ligamentous anterior column at a minimum 1 level); (2) risks of injury to anterior hollow viscus structures, major vessels, and the lumbosacral plexus; (3) the need for 2 approaches, prolonging operative time and risk; (4) complications related to lengthening of the anterior column including stretching of the abdominal aorta; and (5) lack of evidence and familiarity with the procedure.[14–18] Nonetheless, this approach is growing in popularity due to the need for better treatment options.

The concept of MIS has been recently redefined to focus on preserving soft tissue rather than simply limiting skin incision length. Today, the clinical goals of MIS as related to spine surgery include reducing postoperative pain, narcotic consumption, and intraoperative blood loss while at the same time facilitating early mobilization, emphasizing the preservation of functional musculoligamentous structures.[1]

PEDICLE SUBTRACTION OSTEOTOMY

The classic pedicle subtraction osteotomy (PSO) technique was first described by Thomasen in 1985 for the correction of kyphotic deformity.[19] It involves removal of the posterior elements and a wedge-shaped portion of the vertebral body to increase lordosis. PSO enables a correction of up to 30°, which may be required in severe cases of ASD.[3,19] It is ideal for patients with severe fixed angular kyphosis and positive sagittal imbalance greater than 10 cm.[20] Traditional PSO is nevertheless a large open procedure that is subject to all the aforementioned complications associated with open spinal surgery.[21,22] A minimally invasive form of the procedure is, therefore, an attractive alternative to open surgery for achieving a high degree of spinal deformity correction while minimizing perioperative morbidity. PSO offers several advantages over other open and MIS deformity correction techniques, including (1) the ability to treat a completely fused and rigid spine (as with ankylosing spondylitis or in patients who have previously had spinal fusion surgery), (2) the ability to perform the PSO at virtually any level, (3) single position surgery, and (4) widespread spine surgeon familiarity with the technique.

MINI–OPEN PEDICLE SUBTRACTION OSTEOTOMY
Technique

The hybrid mini–open PSO technique was developed to combine the advantages of traditional MIS procedures with those of open surgical deformity correction using PSO.[2] Through this method, a 3-column osteotomy may be performed to correct sagittal plane malalignment. The approach was first explored in a cadaveric model by Voyadzis and colleagues,[20] in 2008, and was first described in vivo by Wang and Madhavan,[1] in 2014. This technique begins with a dorsal skin incision followed by lateral subcutaneous tissue dissection that exposes fascia. Bilateral subperiosteal dissection is then performed at the level of desired PSO, such that the transverse processes are completely exposed and such that the bony exposure extends from the pedicle above to the pedicle below. The spinous process, lamina, and facets of the desired PSO level are subsequently removed and the exiting nerve roots are exposed.

The annulus of the disk space immediately superior to the level of the PSO is cauterized and removed if an extended PSO is desired. The bilateral pedicles are then removed in their entirety. This approach makes the PSO segment an essentially open technique, but because the only subfascial opening is at this 1 level, the morbidity of the soft tissue dissection is similar to an open 1-level posterior fusion. This limited opening, which is much smaller than an open PSO, has 3 major advantages: (1) direct control and inspection of the neural elements at the PSO site, which is potentially at risk, thus enhancing safety; (2) the ability to assemble a construct at the area of greatest lordosis; and (3) the ability to maintain excellent hemostasis.

Next, percutaneous pedicle screws are placed through the fascia, 3 levels above and 3 levels below the PSO level. The extensions of the pedicle screws are used to prevent lateral translation of the vertebral bodies during the osteotomy. For this purpose, 4 lordotic rods are then passed through the screw heads above and below the PSO level bilaterally. Bilateral decancellation osteotomy is subsequently performed to remove 2 cones of cancellous bone from the vertebral body, and the decancellation is extended superiorly into the disk space if an extended PSO is desired. The lateral vertebral body cortical wall is then removed bilaterally in a wedge-shaped pattern matching the decancellation. The posterior vertebral body wall and the posterior longitudinal ligament are then removed by retracting the thecal sac medially and consecutively on each side.

The fusion and fixation caudal to the PSO site are achieved using MIS transforaminal lumbar interbody fusion with interbody cages and possibly with percutaneous iliac screws.[23] Rostral to the PSO level, facet or interlaminar fusions supplement the percutaneous screws. At the site of PSO where the tip of each rod is exposed, a rod-to-rod connector is used to connect each set of rods on either side of midline. Next, set screws

are loosely placed to attach the rods to the screw heads. The rod holders are then carefully forced toward each other creating a greenstick fracture at the osteotomy site. The end result is increased lordosis. The 4-rod technique allows the surgeon to control the osteotomy closure without risking catastrophic translation of the disrupted spinal column. The rod-to-rod connectors are then tightened firmly, followed by tightening of the set screws. **Figs. 1** and **2** illustrate the procedure's ability to correct sagittal and coronal deformity.

Advantages

Mini–open PSO has the advantage of using a cantilever dual-rod construct to maximize the force of correction, particularly in the face of osteoporotic bone.[1] The upper and lower screw-rod constructs on either side act as combined lever units, with the hinge at the anterior portion of the vertebral body. Thus, in contrast to the

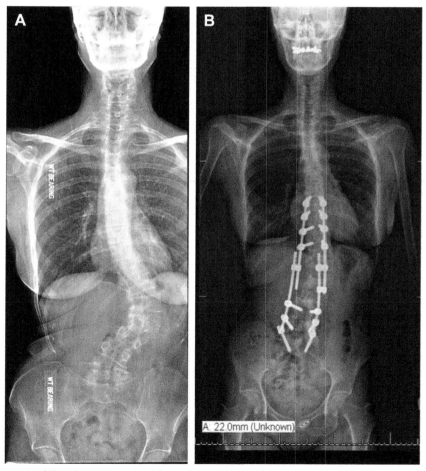

Fig. 1. Preoperative (*A*) and postoperative (*B*) Anteroposterior 36-in standing films demonstrating improvement in scoliosis after mini–open PSO and percutaneous pedicle screw instrumentation.

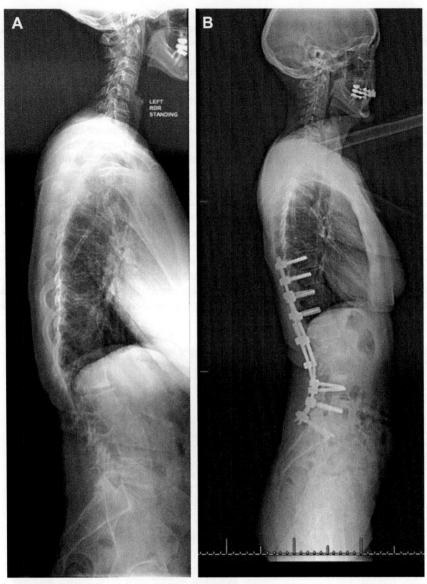

Fig. 2. Preoperative (*A*) and postoperative (*B*) lateral 36-in standing radiographs demonstrating improvement in sagittal alignment after mini–open PSO and percutaneous pedicle screw instrumentation.

traditional segmental correction method at sequential levels, this novel technique allows for forceful correction while minimizing the risk of screw pullout because all the screws connected together by a rod work in unison as 1 unit rather than independently.[2] By opening only the site of PSO, this mini–open technique allows for direct decompression of neural elements and permits direct visualization of the thecal sac during osteotomy closure, which is a potential source of significant complications.[2] Furthermore, this method overcomes the common difficulty of passing a lordotic rod through a kyphotic or flat spine that plagued previous attempts at

significant sagittal deformity correction through minimally invasive means.[23]

Clinical Outcomes and Complications

This hybrid technique has yielded promising results. In a study of 16 patients with ASD treated with mini–open PSO and associated fusion from the thoracic to sacral spine or pelvis, there was improvement in leg visual analog scale (VAS) score, back VAS score, Oswestry Disability Index score, 36-Item Short Form Health Survey (SF-36) physical component summary score, SF-36 mental component summary score, and maximal ambulation distance.[2] In that series, the PSO level was L2 in 38% of cases and L3 in the remaining 62%. Furthermore, there were significant improvements in both coronal and sagittal plane alignment postoperatively. Lumbar lordosis increased by a mean of 25° in all patients. Solid radiographic arthrodesis at all treated levels was achieved in 80% of patients who underwent postoperative CT scanning. Due to the small sample size, definite conclusions regarding complication rates cannot be determined. One patient had an unintentional intraoperative durotomy, 1 patient had a postoperative wound infection, and 1 patient suffered a watershed cerebral stroke secondary to preexisting severe bilateral carotid stenosis. There was 1 iliac screw-rod dislodgement and 1 interbody graft extrusion, both of which required surgical reoperation. Additionally, although there were no cases of pseudarthrosis, there was 1 case (6%) of rod fracture at the PSO site 12 months after surgery. In comparison, the rate of pseudarthrosis and rod fracture in open PSO procedures is approximately 10%.[24] Despite these promising results, sagittal vertical axis less than 60 mm could not be achieved in 3 of the 16 patients who underwent hybrid mini–open PSO.[2] Furthermore, mismatch between lumbar lordosis and pelvic incidence by more than 10° persisted in 4 cases. Another drawback of the hybrid mini–open PSO technique is that it relies heavily on the off-label use of cages and osteobiologics to promote fusion.[2]

SUMMARY

The correction of sagittal and coronal deformity is a complicated endeavor that carries a high risk of complications. The MIS PSO approach was developed to overcome some of the drawbacks and risks of open surgery while maintaining the versatility of the PSO procedure. More clinical and radiographic evidence is needed, however, to further validate the approach compared with other, more widely studied, operations.

REFERENCES

1. Wang MY, Madhavan K. Mini-open pedicle subtraction osteotomy: surgical technique. World Neurosurg 2014;81(5-6):843.e11-4.
2. Wang MY, Bordon G. Mini-open pedicle subtraction osteotomy as a treatment for severe adult spinal deformities: case series with initial clinical and radiographic outcomes. J Neurosurg Spine 2016;24(5):769–76.
3. Heary RF, Bono CM. Pedicle subtraction osteotomy in the treatment of chronic, posttraumatic kyphotic deformity. J Neurosurg Spine 2006;5(1):1–8.
4. Kim YJ, Bridwell KH, Lenke LG, et al. Results of lumbar pedicle subtraction osteotomies for fixed sagittal imbalance: a minimum 5-year follow-up study. Spine (Phila Pa 1976) 2007;32(20):2189–97.
5. Mummaneni PV, Dhall SS, Ondra SL, et al. Pedicle subtraction osteotomy. Neurosurgery 2008;63(3 Suppl):171–6.
6. Smith JS, Shaffrey CI, Glassman SD, et al. Risk-benefit assessment of surgery for adult scoliosis: an analysis based on patient age. Spine (Phila Pa 1976) 2011;36(10):817–24.
7. Weistroffer JK, Perra JH, Lonstein JE, et al. Complications in long fusions to the sacrum for adult scoliosis: minimum five-year analysis of fifty patients. Spine (Phila Pa 1976) 2008;33(13):1478–83.
8. Charosky S, Guigui P, Blamoutier A, et al, Study Group on Scoliosis. Complications and risk factors of primary adult scoliosis surgery: a multicenter study of 306 patients. Spine (Phila Pa 1976) 2012; 37(8):693–700.
9. Haque RM, Mundis GM Jr, Ahmed Y, et al. Comparison of radiographic results after minimally invasive, hybrid, and open surgery for adult spinal deformity: a multicenter study of 184 patients. Neurosurg Focus 2014;36(5):E13.
10. Schwender JD, Holly LT, Rouben DP, et al. Minimally invasive transforaminal lumbar interbody fusion (TLIF): technical feasibility and initial results. J Spinal Disord Tech 2005;18(Suppl):S1–6.
11. Acosta FL, Liu J, Slimack N, et al. Changes in coronal and sagittal plane alignment following minimally invasive direct lateral interbody fusion for the treatment of degenerative lumbar disease in adults: a radiographic study. J Neurosurg Spine 2011;15(1):92–6.
12. Karikari IO, Nimjee SM, Hardin CA, et al. Extreme lateral interbody fusion approach for isolated thoracic and thoracolumbar spine diseases: initial clinical experience and early outcomes. J Spinal Disord Tech 2011;24(6):368–75.
13. Costanzo G, Zoccali C, Maykowski P, et al. The role of minimally invasive lateral lumbar interbody fusion in sagittal balance correction and spinal deformity. Eur Spine J 2014;23(Suppl 6):699–704.
14. Turner JD, Akbarnia BA, Eastlack RK, et al. Radiographic outcomes of anterior column realignment for adult sagittal plane deformity: a multicenter analysis. Eur Spine J 2015;24(Suppl 3):427–32.
15. Marchi L, Pimenta L, Oliveira L, et al. Distance between great vessels and the lumbar spine: MRI study for anterior longitudinal ligament release through a lateral approach. J Neurol Surg A Cent Eur Neurosurg 2017;78(2):144–53.
16. Deukmedjian A, Uribe JS. Minimally invasive anterior column reconstruction for sagittal plane deformities. In: Wang M, Lu Y, Anderson D, et al, editors. Minimally invasive spinal deformity surgery. Vienna (Austria): Springer; 2014. p. 273–86.

17. Deukmedjian AR, Dakwar E, Ahmadian A, et al. Early outcomes of minimally invasive anterior longitudinal ligament release for correction of sagittal imbalance in patients with adult spinal deformity. ScientificWorldJournal 2012;2012:789698.

18. Akbarnia BA, Mundis GM Jr, Moazzaz P, et al. Anterior column realignment (ACR) for focal kyphotic spinal deformity using a lateral transpsoas approach and ALL release. J Spinal Disord Tech 2014;27(1): 29–39.

19. Thomasen E. Vertebral osteotomy for correction of kyphosis in ankylosing spondylitis. Clin Orthop Relat Res 1985;(194):142–52.

20. Voyadzis JM, Gala VC, O'Toole JE, et al. Minimally invasive posterior osteotomies. Neurosurgery 2008; 63(3 Suppl):204–10.

21. Bridwell KH, Lewis SJ, Edwards C, et al. Complications and outcomes of pedicle subtraction osteotomies for fixed sagittal imbalance. Spine (Phila Pa 1976) 2003;28(18):2093–101.

22. Yang BP, Ondra SL, Chen LA, et al. Clinical and radiographic outcomes of thoracic and lumbar pedicle subtraction osteotomy for fixed sagittal imbalance. J Neurosurg Spine 2006;5(1):9–17.

23. Wang MY. Miniopen pedicle subtraction osteotomy: surgical technique and initial results. Neurosurg Clin N Am 2014;25(2):347–51.

24. Dickson DD, Lenke LG, Bridwell KH, et al. Risk factors for and assessment of symptomatic pseudarthrosis after lumbar pedicle subtraction osteotomy in adult spinal deformity. Spine (Phila Pa 1976) 2014; 39(15):1190–5.

The Challenge of the Lumbosacral Fractional Curve in the Setting of Adult Degenerative Scoliosis

Peter G. Campbell, MD*, Pierce D. Nunley, MD

KEYWORDS

- Fractional curve • Scoliosis • Fusion • Scoliosis correction • Adult degenerative scoliosis
- L5 obliquity • Adult spinal deformity

KEY POINTS

- In the setting of adult degenerative scoliosis (ADS), the compensatory curve at the level of the lumbosacral junction below the major curve is called the fractional curve.
- The L4, L5, and S1 nerve roots on the side of the concavity of the fractional curve are the most frequent radicular pain generators in the setting of ADS.
- Ending a scoliosis construct at L4 or L5 with a preexisting the fractional curve places patients at high risk of adjacent segment breakdown or causing a compensatory major curve above the correction.
- Instrumentation options to address the fractional curve include anterior lumbar interbody fusion, oblique lumbar interbody fusion, posterior or transforaminal lumbar interbody fusion, and open rod reduction techniques.

INTRODUCTION

Adult degenerative scoliosis (ADS) is a 3-dimensional spinal disorder affecting the skeletally mature adult spine. Epidemiologically, degenerative lumbar scoliosis primarily involves patients in the sixth decade of life or greater, with a female predilection. ADS is thought to be related to osteoporotic degeneration and/or degenerative disk disease resulting in an asymmetric degradation of the intervertebral disk and facet joints.[1,2] These distortions induce a progressive lateral listhesis or rotation of the vertebra and ultimately lead to scoliosis, loss of lumbar lordosis, vertebral body translation, and rotational subluxation.[3]

In treating ADS, the main indication for performing an instrumented fusion is a lumbar curve. Unlike the typical adolescent patient with scoliosis, the curve parameters are generally considered to be unsuitable for ending fixation at L3 or L4.[4] Oftentimes, a rotatory subluxation or a coronal imbalance is present at the L4 or L5 segments. In the setting of ADS, the compensatory curve at the level of the lumbosacral junction below the major curve is called the fractional curve.[5]

The general goals of adult deformity surgery mirror those of the adolescent population in that the goals are to obtain sagittal and coronal balance, symptom relief, and solid fusion.[6,7] However, one of the difficulties in attempting to apply minimally invasive techniques to ADS curves has been in the treatment of the fractional curve.[5] Traditional approaches to deformity correction of degenerative lumbar scoliosis include both anterior-posterior approaches as well as posterior-only treatments. Open surgical procedures allow the surgeon to

Disclosure Statement: Consultant: 4 Web (P.G. Campbell). Royalties: K2M, LDR. Speakers bureau: K2M, LDR. Consultant: K2M. Stock: Amedica, Paradigm, Spineology (P.D. Nunley).
Spine Institute of Louisiana, 1500 Line Avenue, Shreveport, LA 71101, USA
* Corresponding author.
E-mail address: pcampbell@louisianaspine.org

perform specific techniques that create spinal destabilization to ultimately facilitate correction of the deformity. Minimally invasive spinal surgery offers fewer options for rigid curve manipulation at the lumbosacral junctions and the successful surgeon must evaluate the fractional curve preoperatively to ensure adherence to these established goals to prevent clinical decline secondary to the complication of spinopelvic malalignment.

CHALLENGES IN TREATING THE FRACTIONAL CURVE

In treating ADS, full-length standing anteroposterior and lateral radiographs are obtained to identify spinopelvic parameters. A detailed discussion of correction of these parameters is outside the scope of this article and will be addressed elsewhere in this publication. Typically ADS curves have a lumbar apex.[8] These deformities often are

associated with lumbar hypolordosis and distal reciprocating curves without significant scoliosis in the upper thoracic levels. A fractional curve, L4 to the sacrum, is often appreciated on anteroposterior imaging (**Fig. 1**).

Much like other degenerative conditions, pain is the indication for seeking treatment for more than 90% of the ADS patient population.[9] Patients with ADS may present with back pain associated with scoliotic curve progression or neurologic symptoms, including radiculopathy and central stenosis.[10] Severe foraminal stenosis is present in up to 97% of patients with ADS on radiographical evaluation.[11] Furthermore, the prevalence of radicular pain has been demonstrated to be significantly increased at the levels of the caudal nerve roots. The probability of radiculopathy has been shown to increase in a linear fashion as the level of the root advances caudally.[12] Hence, the L4, L5, and S1 nerve roots on the side of the concavity

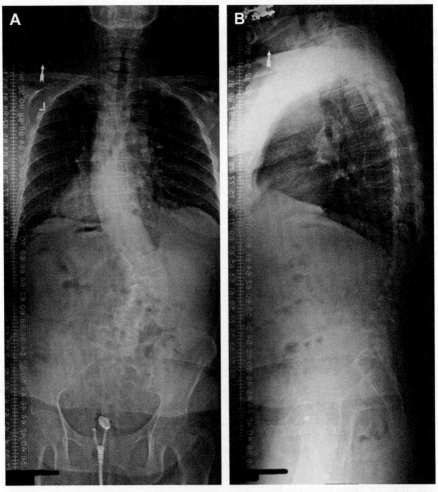

Fig. 1. (*A*) Anteroposterior and (*B*) lateral 36-inch standing radiographs demonstrating an ADS major curve with an apex at the L2/3 disk space and a fractional curve causing a rightward obliquity of L5.

of the fractional curve are the most frequent radicular pain generators in the setting of ADS.[2]

Over the past 70 years, spinal deformity surgeons have developed an extensive understanding of the principal tenets and goals of open surgical intervention.[5] In recent years, the prevailing dogma from this discipline has been that appropriate alignment of the sagittal plane has the greatest bearing on long-term patient outcomes.[13,14] As a piquant corollary, coronal balance has largely been deemphasized in the ADS population.[12] Given that the presence of neurologic symptoms and deficits has been strongly correlated with the decision to pursue operative treatment of ADS, spine surgeons must include in their surgical planning the symptomatic radicular levels that are more frequently relatable to the fractional (caudal) curve than major lumbar curve.[12,15]

In treating ADS, spine surgeons must weigh the extent of surgical intervention against inevitably increasing the rate of complications associated with length of the surgical construct. Although there is no consensus regarding the best available option, decompression alone; direct or indirect decompression with short-segment fusion; and long-segment fusions are frequently used.[16,17] If short-segment fusion is selected, degeneration can be accelerated in the remaining curve and result in adjacent segment disease.[17] Therefore, to theoretically reduce or avoid adjacent segment pathology, a long fusion extending from the thoracic spine to the sacrum may be performed. However, this invariably increases both the major complication rate as well as unplanned reoperation rate in this elderly population.[18]

Ending a surgical construct before the lumbosacral junction in ADS often occurs when a surgeon is attempting to minimize the number of levels fused and thus the complication rate of the index surgery. Maintenance of motion at the L4/5 or L5/S1 segments does allow for the innate pelvic compensatory mobility to accommodate a stiff construct above the lumbosacral junction.[19] However, the most common complication with stopping fusion at L4 or L5 seems to be adjacent segment disease at the L5/S1 disk.[20] Literature-reported rates of adjacent segment disease at L5-S1 after short and long-segment ADS fusions range from 38% to 61%.[21–24] One factor that has been isolated as potentially placing patients at high risk for adjacent segment breakdown after fusions ending at L4 or L5 is the presence of a preexisting fractional curve at L5/S1.[5] Ending a construct above a fractional curve makes subsequent spinal balance difficult to achieve, while also making it more likely that any adjacent segment degeneration will lead to a decreasing cross-sectional area in one foramen.

Postoperatively, this may lead to a clinically symptomatic L5 radiculopathy that could ultimately require a revision surgery requiring extension to the sacrum.[4] Some investigators have recommended that all fractional curves greater than 15° must be corrected and included within the construct.[8]

Consideration and management of the fractional curve at L5 is of paramount importance in treating patients with ADS with fusion techniques. If a fractional curve is present and is not addressed at the time of the index surgery, the patient is very unlikely to ever obtain appropriate coronal balance.[25] If a minimally invasive solution is selected, surgeons must understand and be able to realistically gauge the degree of obtainable correction.[5] In ADS, rigid fractional curves are generally recommended to be included in the fusion construct and often require management with interbody cage placement to prevent coronal decompensation[25] (**Fig. 2**).

CHALLENGES MANAGING THE LUMBOSACRAL JUNCTION IN ADULT DEGENERATIVE SCOLIOSIS

There remains considerable controversy in the literature regarding the distal fusion level for ADS in the setting of a long construct fusion.[20] However, there seems to be a consensus on several situations whereby fixation to the sacrum seems to be necessary. Many spine surgeons agree that indications to include the sacrum in an ADS construct include the presence of an L5/S1 spondylolisthesis, if an L5 or S1 radiculopathy is present, decompression at the L5/S1 segment has been previously done, and the presence of a fractional curve at the lumbosacral junction (**Box 1**).[4,19,20] On the other hand, terminating a long-segment fusion at L5 when the L5/S1 segment is healthy can be useful to maintaining lumbar motion, reduce operative morbidity, and decrease perioperative complication rates associated with lumbosacral fixation.[19] However, disadvantages to L4 or L5 construct termination include the increased potential for adjacent segment degeneration at L5/S1, loss of ability to correct sagittal plane deformities with the index operation, and the lack of a solid fixation endpoint for pedicle screw fixation owing to the L5 pedicle anatomy and its higher cross-sectional cancellous bone content.[4,19] If there is a substantial amount of degeneration at L5/S1, most surgeons would likely advocate for fusing to the sacrum in the setting of scoliosis[4]; however, considerable disagreement exists as to how to assess the amount of degeneration radiographically. On plain radiographs, validated algorithms exist that score disk degeneration by

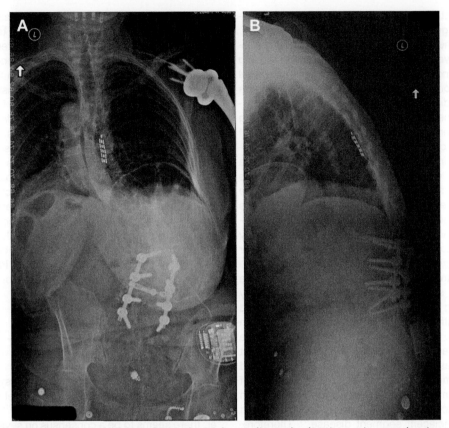

Fig. 2. (*A*) Anteroposterior and (*B*) lateral 36-inch standing radiographs showing an increased major curve after L3-S1 fusion without correction of the fractional curve.

evaluating variables such as disk height, status of the end plates, spondylolisthesis, and vacuum disk phenomenon.[26] Scoring the L5/S1 disk in the setting of ADS on radiographic evaluation is quite difficult given any obliquity and opacification related to pelvic structures. The use of MRI to evaluate disk degeneration has not been validated for this indication.[27] Furthermore, the use of MRI to evaluate disk degeneration in this setting is plagued with difficulties such as poor correlates between mild and moderate disk disease to pain,

lack of a clear clinical correlation of Modic endplate changes to pain, and the interobserver variability of assessing the disk itself in the setting of coexistant lumbar scolosis.[4,28] Computed tomography scans have been used to evaluate for facet arthropathy at this level with uncertain significance given that patients in the age range necessary to acquire ADS often have degenerative changes.[29] Even if there is only minor degeneration in the L5/S1 disk, for patients with a sagittal imbalance and lumbar hypolordosis, most investigators agree that the L5-S1 segment should be included in the fusion to attempt to correct these parameters of global spinal alignment.[4,20,30]

Several clinical challenges exist in the ADS patient population when considering a longer construct fusion to include the fractional curve. Consideration of correction of both coronal and sagittal plane deformity often requires long posterior constructs from the distal thoracic spine to the sacrum. Given the long lever arms and associated cantilever forces, high amounts of stress are placed on the base of the construct.[31] Additionally, cancellous L5 and S1 pedicles coupled with osteopenia and osteoporosis in the elderly patient may

---

Box 1
Indications to fuse to sacrum in a long-segment construct for adult degenerative scoliosis

Spondylolisthesis at L5/S1

Pars defects at L5

Central stenosis at L5/S1

Symptomatic radiculopathy of L5 or S1 nerve roots

Prior laminectomy at L5/S1

L5/S1 obliquity (fractional curve)

lead to distal hardware failure. Common techniques to augment long-segment fusions for additional sacropelvic fixation include the use of S2 alar iliac screws and iliac bolts.[32] The addition of these types of pelvic fixation provides the attractive biomechanical profile of being both divergent anchors from the proximal fixation points in the coronal plane as well as a stabilization point anterior to the axis of rotation of the pelvis to help further resist distal pullout.[32,33] Although absolute and relative indications for using this instrumentation remain undefined, these contemporary pelvic fixation techniques offer an improved construct profile for long-segment fusion that reduces distal failure in at-risk patients.[31]

TECHNIQUES TO CORRECT THE FRACTIONAL CURVE

The stated goals of adult deformity surgery are to obtain sagittal and coronal balance, symptom relief, and solid fusion.[6,7] However, the ADS population is often elderly and prone to higher perioperative complications. A recent multicenter prospective study conducted to assess perioperative and postoperative complication rates after open ADS procedures identified a 69.8% complication rate at 2-year follow-up. Furthermore, 28.2% of patients required 1 or more reoperations.[34] Given the high complication rates of this procedure, treatment goals are often adjusted to focus more on symptom management as an important subcontext of the overall scoliosis surgical planning.[35] To this end, various techniques to achieve preoperative planning goals have been described in the literature.[36] Decompression alone at the level of radiculopathy is occasionally used to treat severe radiculopathy. Placement of interbody cages that aide in the correction of deformity, and provide anterior column support and circumferential arthrodesis are often described as viable options. Furthermore, short-segment and long-segment posterior instrumentation with facetectomies have also been used for more extensive deformity correction. All the previously described strategies have been used to treat fractional curve pathology.

ADS treatment is a challenge for spine surgeons especially when treating an elderly patient population with multiple medical comorbidities whereby corrective operations may result in prohibitively high complication rates. Oftentimes the presenting complaint is severe radiculopathy, which has been shown to occur more frequently at the level of the caudal nerve roots. This often necessitates treatment of the fractional curve.[2] Various minimally invasive decompressions involving the use of microscopes, tubular retractors, and endoscopes have been developed to treat this type of degenerative disease. These techniques largely focus on the preservation of the posterior elements, supraspinous and intraspinous ligaments, and facet joints.[37] Literature regarding decompression alone for ADS often does not support decompression to provide successful longer-term outcomes.[3,38,39] However, some investigators do offer decompression alone as an option in certain settings. Berven and colleagues[40] suggest a unilateral minimally invasive spine (MIS) decompression for patients with ADS with radicular pain only stemming from the convex side of the deformity with an intact pars interarticularis and facet joint. Hansraj and colleagues[41] reported that decompression alone could be performed in patients with central stenosis and less than 20° of coronal curvature. Kato and colleagues[37] noted poor success rates if MIS decompression is performed at a level with greater than 3° of coronal disk wedging or lateral listhesis at the treated level. This was noted to be especially severe if it occurred at the level of the L4/5 space. Other investigators have also found that similar radiographic findings alone were strong predictors of progression of a degenerative scoliosis curve.[42] Using an MIS decompression in the fractional curve has been presented in the literature as an option in very select cases when there are no signs of asymmetrical degeneration that would predispose patients to postoperative curve progression and thus an extensive reconstructive procedure.

Spine surgeons performing scoliosis operations generally pay close attention to the lumbosacral junction. Anterior lumbar interbody fusion (ALIF) is often used to address the clinical symptoms associated with a fractional curve at L4/5 and L5/S1. ALIF has been considered the gold standard technique for interbody fusion.[43] ALIF provides several benefits in the setting of ADS: (1) large graft size with significant surface area for fusion, (2) anterior load sharing with the posterior hardware, (3) indirect decompression of a narrowed neural foramen in the fractional curve, (4) sectioning of the anterior longitudinal ligament, which allows for increased lordosis to be added to the final construct, and (5) improved coronal and sagittal balance.[5] An L4/5 and L5/S1 ALIF at the base of a long-segment scoliosis construct will effectively address the fractional curve in its entirety. In a review by McPhee and Swanson,[44] staged anterior and posterior lumbar procedures showed better fractional curve improvement as well as sagittal balance correction in patients with ADS than posterior procedures alone. Unfortunately, the addition of ALIF to a scoliosis solution is also associated with disadvantages, including increased intraoperative time and anesthetic times, the risk of intra-abdominal vascular and visceral injury, as well as superior hypogastric plexus injury.[36,45]

Minimally invasive techniques have recently been applied to surgical correction of ADS.[46] When treating a disease process endemic to an aging population, the reduction of tissue dissection and perioperative complications rates is certainly paramount. Access to the L5/S1 space is currently problematic for traditional transpsoas procedures currently used for lateral access. Hence, with this traditional transpsoas approach, there is often a need for another surgical approach to fully treat the fractional curve.[47] A second lateral technique first described in 2012, called a prepsoas approach for an oblique lumbar interbody fusion (OLIF), has been suggested as a possibly less invasive option to provide fractional curve stability at the lumbosacral junction.[48] Although this procedure is discussed elsewhere in this issue in full detail, this approach has been publicized as a potential option to obtain access of multiple lumbar interspaces, including both the L4/5 and L5/S1 levels, with an anterior fusion corridor associated with potentially fewer complications than direct lateral transpsoas approaches.[49] The theoretic benefit of the prepsoas OLIF is the ability to manipulate the fractional curve in both the coronal and sagittal planes through 1 minimally invasive incision. However, it still shares the associated risks of the ALIF operation, such as increased operative times and vascular injury. Current literature has not fully critically evaluated the indications for the prepsoas OLIF procedure in the setting of spinal deformity at this time.

Interbody cages placed through a posterior approach are also options when attempting to correct a fractional curve. The posterior insertion of rigid cages can restore the disk height and possibly provide a mechanism for lasting decompression of the neural elements. Using a unilateral interbody cage insertion, Heary and colleagues[7] reported excellent improvements in coronal imbalance in patients with ADS when a unilateral interbody cage was inserted into the concavity of the curve. Wang[47] reported an improvement in both the coronal and sagittal alignment with unilateral insertion of an expandable mesh bag. Wang[47] suggested placement of a unilaterally inserted cage into the side of the concavity of the fractional curve to elevate and correct the curve. However, posteriorly inserted interbody cages do require more extensive bony resection than posterior surgery alone, an increased operative time for facetectomy and discectomy, and a narrow access corridor mandates a smaller implant footprint that can result in postoperative subsidence.[43]

Unlike adolescent scoliosis, fractional curves in ASD are generally associated with a rigid spine. Hence, open surgical approaches may be more powerful in obtaining sagittal alignment; however, at the cost of increased perioperative complication rates. Posterior techniques to provide a correction of the fractional curve can be used. This includes both osteotomy and rod reduction options. Rod rotation maneuvers allow the frontal scoliotic deformity to be converted into a lumbar lordosis with a 3-dimensional correction.[50] However, these techniques are limited by anterior or lateral bridging osteophytes that can be released only by a circumferential surgical option.[51]

SUMMARY

Understanding the relationship of the lumbosacral fractional curve to degenerative scoliosis is critically important to surgical management. Likewise, it is vitally important for surgeons to understand the etiology and pathogenesis of this disease process, given the increasing patient age as well as the resultant associated increase in medical comorbidities experienced with large corrective operations. As more minimally invasive instrumentation solutions are applied to ADS to decrease perioperative complication rates, surgeons must realize that ending a construct at an L5 obliquity may ultimately lead to suboptimal patient outcomes.[5] Whereas a well-planned ALIF procedure effectively corrects the fractional curve, other prepsoas oblique MIS and open posterior treatment strategies continue to be options available to the contemporary spine surgeon.

The latest generation of spinal reconstructive instruments and implants allows for very powerful 3-dimensional multipoint correction of deformity. This allows the forces to be distributed to multiple fixation points, decreasing implant failure and allowing for safe correction of significant deformities even in the presence of osteoporosis, which is a frequent comorbidity in this population. Many of these techniques have recently been modified for use in minimally invasive surgery. With every new technology there are nuances and techniques that are not necessarily intuitively or deductively obvious. Therefore, it is vital for surgeons learning new techniques to obtain appropriate knowledge and training. Although many resources are available, mentoring remains the best way to assimilate new techniques. Visiting a surgeon skilled in the technique being sought is recommended by the authors.

We are continually learning more about how to treat ASD and what parameters and techniques are appropriate for each specific patient. With the advent of institutional research and prospective registries, we will be able to continue to improve techniques and case selection to provide guidance for surgical planning and execution to provide the best care for our patients into the future.

REFERENCES

1. Daffner SD, Vaccaro AR. Adult degenerative lumbar scoliosis. Am J Orthop (Belle Mead NJ) 2003;32(2): 77–82 [discussion: 82].
2. Ploumis A, Transfeldt EE, Gilbert TJ, et al. Radiculopathy in degenerative lumbar scoliosis: correlation of stenosis with relief from selective nerve root steroid injections. Pain Med 2011;12(1):45–50.
3. Aebi M. The adult scoliosis. Eur Spine J 2005; 14(10):925–48.
4. Bridwell KH, Edwards CC, Lenke LG. The pros and cons to saving the L5-S1 motion segment in a long scoliosis fusion construct. Spine (Phila Pa 1976) 2003;28(20):S234–42.
5. Wang MY. The importance of the fractional curve. In: Wang MY, Lu Y, Anderson GD, et al, editors. Minimally invasive spinal deformity surgery: an evolution of modern techniques. Vienna: Springer; 2014. p. 47–52.
6. Birknes JK, White AP, Albert TJ, et al. Adult degenerative scoliosis: a review. Neurosurgery 2008;63(3 Suppl):94–103.
7. Heary RF, Kumar S, Bono CM. Decision making in adult deformity. Neurosurgery 2008;63(3 Suppl):69–77.
8. Silva FE, Lenke LG. Adult degenerative scoliosis: evaluation and management. Neurosurg Focus 2010;28(3):E1.
9. Winter RB, Lonstein JE, Denis F. Pain patterns in adult scoliosis. Orthop Clin North Am 1988;19(2):339–45.
10. Schwab FJ, Smith VA, Biserni M, et al. Adult scoliosis: a quantitative radiographic and clinical analysis. Spine (Phila Pa 1976) 2002;27(4):387–92.
11. Fu KM, Rhagavan P, Shaffrey CI, et al. Prevalence, severity, and impact of foraminal and canal stenosis among adults with degenerative scoliosis. Neurosurgery 2011;69(6):1181–7.
12. Hawasli AH, Chang J, Yarbrough CK, et al. Interpedicular height as a predictor of radicular pain in adult degenerative scoliosis. Spine J 2016;16(9): 1070–8.
13. Glassman SD, Bridwell K, Dimar JR, et al. The impact of positive sagittal balance in adult spinal deformity. Spine (Phila Pa 1976) 2005;30(18):2024–9.
14. Schwab F, Lafage V, Patel A, et al. Sagittal plane considerations and the pelvis in the adult patient. Spine (Phila Pa 1976) 2009;34(17):1828–33.
15. Smith JS, Shaffrey CI, Berven S, et al. Operative versus nonoperative treatment of leg pain in adults with scoliosis: a retrospective review of a prospective multicenter database with two-year follow-up. Spine (Phila Pa 1976) 2009;34(16):1693–8.
16. Bridwell KH. Selection of instrumentation and fusion levels for scoliosis: where to start and where to stop.

Invited submission from the Joint Section Meeting on Disorders of the Spine and Peripheral Nerves, March 2004. J Neurosurg Spine 2004;1(1):1–8.
17. Cho KJ, Suk SI, Park SR, et al. Short fusion versus long fusion for degenerative lumbar scoliosis. Eur Spine J 2008;17(5):650–6.
18. Akbarnia BA, Ogilvie JW, Hammerberg KW. Debate: degenerative scoliosis: to operate or not to operate. Spine (Phila Pa 1976) 2006;31(19 Suppl):S195–201.
19. Swamy G, Berven SH, Bradford DS. The selection of L5 versus S1 in long fusions for adult idiopathic scoliosis. Neurosurg Clin N Am 2007;18(2):281–8.
20. Cho KJ, Suk SI, Park SR, et al. Arthrodesis to L5 versus S1 in long instrumentation and fusion for degenerative lumbar scoliosis. Eur Spine J 2009; 18(4):531–7.
21. Edwards CC, Bridwell KH, Patel A, et al. Long adult deformity fusions to L5 and the sacrum. A matched cohort analysis. Spine (Phila Pa 1976) 2004;29(18): 1996–2005.
22. Edwards CC, Bridwell KH, Patel A, et al. Thoracolumbar deformity arthrodesis to L5 in adults: the fate of the L5-S1 disc. Spine (Phila Pa 1976) 2003; 28(18):2122–31.
23. Emami A, Deviren V, Berven S, et al. Outcome and complications of long fusions to the sacrum in adult spine deformity: Luque-Galveston, combined iliac and sacral screws, and sacral fixation. Spine (Phila Pa 1976) 2002;27(7):776–86.
24. Horton WC, Holt RT, Muldowny DS. Controversy. Fusion of L5-S1 in adult scoliosis. Spine (Phila Pa 1976) 1996;21(21):2520–2.
25. Youssef JA, Orndorff DO, Patty CA, et al. Current status of adult spinal deformity. Global Spine J 2013;3(1):51–62.
26. Weiner DK, Distell B, Studenski S, et al. Does radiographic osteoarthritis correlate with flexibility of the lumbar spine? J Am Geriatr Soc 1994;42(3):257–63.
27. Pfirrmann CW, Metzdorf A, Zanetti M, et al. Magnetic resonance classification of lumbar intervertebral disc degeneration. Spine (Phila Pa 1976) 2001;26(17): 1873–8.
28. Sandhu HS, Sanchez-Caso LP, Parvataneni HK, et al. Association between findings of provocative discography and vertebral endplate signal changes as seen on MRI. J Spinal Disord 2000;13(5):438–43.
29. Boos N, Weissbach S, Rohrbach H, et al. Classification of age-related changes in lumbar intervertebral discs: 2002 Volvo Award in basic science. Spine (Phila Pa 1976) 2002;27(23):2631–44.
30. Schwab FJ, Blondel B, Bess S, et al. Radiographical spinopelvic parameters and disability in the setting of adult spinal deformity: a prospective multicenter analysis. Spine (Phila Pa 1976) 2013;38(13):E803–12.
31. Shen FH, Mason JR, Shimer AL, et al. Pelvic fixation for adult scoliosis. Eur Spine J 2013;22(Suppl 2): S265–75.

32. Kebaish KM. Sacropelvic fixation: techniques and complications. Spine (Phila Pa 1976) 2010;35(25): 2245–51.

33. McCord DH, Cunningham BW, Shono Y, et al. Biomechanical analysis of lumbosacral fixation. Spine (Phila Pa 1976) 1992;17(8 Suppl):S235–43.

34. Smith JS, Klineberg E, Lafage V, et al. Prospective multicenter assessment of perioperative and minimum 2-year postoperative complication rates associated with adult spinal deformity surgery. J Neurosurg Spine 2016;25(1):1–14.

35. Turner JA, Ersek M, Herron L, et al. Surgery for lumbar spinal stenosis. Attempted meta-analysis of the literature. Spine (Phila Pa 1976) 1992; 17(1):1–8.

36. Mobbs RJ, Phan K, Malham G, et al. Lumbar interbody fusion: techniques, indications and comparison of interbody fusion options including PLIF, TLIF, MI-TLIF, OLIF/ATP, LLIF and ALIF. J Spine Surg 2015;1(1):2–18.

37. Kato M, Namikawa T, Matsumura A, et al. Radiographic risk factors of reoperation following minimally invasive decompression for lumbar canal stenosis associated with degenerative scoliosis and spondylolisthesis. Glob Spine J 2017;7(6): 498–505.

38. Frazier DD, Lipson SJ, Fossel AH, et al. Associations between spinal deformity and outcomes after decompression for spinal stenosis. Spine (Phila Pa 1976) 1997;22(17):2025–9.

39. Vaccaro AR, Ball ST. Indications for instrumentation in degenerative lumbar spinal disorders. Orthopedics 2000;23(3):260–71 [quiz: 272–263].

40. Berven SH, Deviren V, Mitchell B, et al. Operative management of degenerative scoliosis: an evidence-based approach to surgical strategies based on clinical and radiographic outcomes. Neurosurg Clin N Am 2007;18(2):261–72.

41. Hansraj KK, O'Leary PF, Cammisa FP, et al. Decompression, fusion, and instrumentation surgery for complex lumbar spinal stenosis. Clin Orthop Relat Res 2001;(384):18–25.

42. Seo JY, Ha KY, Hwang TH, et al. Risk of progression of degenerative lumbar scoliosis. J Neurosurg Spine 2011;15(5):558–66.

43. Yen CP, Mosley YI, Uribe JS. Role of minimally invasive surgery for adult spinal deformity in preventing complications. Curr Rev Musculoskelet Med 2016; 9(3):309–15.

44. McPhee IB, Swanson CE. The surgical management of degenerative lumbar scoliosis. Posterior instrumentation alone versus two stage surgery. Bull Hosp Jt Dis 1998;57(1):16–22.

45. Phan K, Thayaparan GK, Mobbs RJ. Anterior lumbar interbody fusion versus transforaminal lumbar interbody fusion–systematic review and meta-analysis. Br J Neurosurg 2015;29(5):705–11.

46. Anand N, Baron EM. Minimally invasive approaches for the correction of adult spinal deformity. Eur Spine J 2013;22(Suppl 2):S232–41.

47. Wang MY. Improvement of sagittal balance and lumbar lordosis following less invasive adult spinal deformity surgery with expandable cages and percutaneous instrumentation. J Neurosurg Spine 2013;18(1):4–12.

48. Silvestre C, Mac-Thiong JM, Hilmi R, et al. Complications and morbidities of mini-open anterior retroperitoneal lumbar interbody fusion: oblique lumbar interbody fusion in 179 patients. Asian Spine J 2012;6(2):89–97.

49. Mehren C, Mayer HM, Zandanell C, et al. The oblique anterolateral approach to the lumbar spine provides access to the lumbar spine with few early complications. Clin Orthop Relat Res 2016;474(9):2020–7.

50. Matsumura A, Namikawa T, Kato M, et al. Posterior corrective surgery with a multilevel transforaminal lumbar interbody fusion and a rod rotation maneuver for patients with degenerative lumbar kyphoscoliosis. J Neurosurg Spine 2017;26(2):150–7.

51. Hsieh MK, Chen LH, Niu CC, et al. Combined anterior lumbar interbody fusion and instrumented posterolateral fusion for degenerative lumbar scoliosis: indication and surgical outcomes. BMC Surg 2015;15:26.

Moving?

Make sure your subscription moves with you!

To notify us of your new address, find your **Clinics Account Number** (located on your mailing label above your name), and contact customer service at:

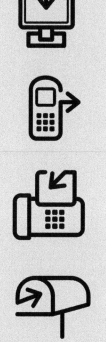

Email: journalscustomerservice-usa@elsevier.com

800-654-2452 (subscribers in the U.S. & Canada)
314-447-8871 (subscribers outside of the U.S. & Canada)

Fax number: 314-447-8029

Elsevier Health Sciences Division
Subscription Customer Service
3251 Riverport Lane
Maryland Heights, MO 63043

ELSEVIER

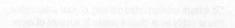

Printed and bound by CPI Group (UK) Ltd, Croydon, CR0 4YY

08/05/2025

01864729-0002